CONCEIVING LUC

CONCEIVING LUC

A Family Story

Liza Freilicher and Jennifer Scheu
with Suzanne Wetanson

WILLIAM MORROW AND COMPANY, INC.

NEW YORK

All the names in *Conceiving Luc,* except for those of family members,
Hilary Steele, and Steven Donziger, have been changed
to protect the privacy of those involved.

It is the policy of William Morrow and Company, Inc., and its imprints
and affiliates, recognizing the importance of preserving what has been written,
to print the books we publish on acid-free paper,
and we exert our best efforts to that end.

Library of Congress Cataloging-in-Publication Data
Freilicher, Liza.
Conceiving Luc : a family story / Liza Freilicher and Jennifer
Scheu ; with Suzanne Wetanson.
p.   cm.
ISBN 0-688-15986-9
1. Surrogate motherhood—Case studies.   2. Surrogate motherhood—
Psychological aspects.   I. Scheu, Jennifer.   II. Wetanson,
Suzanne.   III. Title.
HQ759.5.F74   1999
306.874'3—dc21   98-52060
CIP

Printed in the United States of America
First Edition
1 2 3 4 5 6 7 8 9 10

BOOK DESIGN BY OKSANA KUSHNIR

www.williammorrow.com

FOR LAURIE

ACKNOWLEDGMENTS

First and foremost, I thank my beautiful cousin Jennifer. Simply, she is the most incredible person I have ever known. Her love, kindness, strength, selflessness, and courage have given us the most magical gift of life; without her there would be no "conceiving Luc." She has always been and will always be a person the world and I will admire for everything that she is and her amazing contributions.

My loving mother and best friend, Suzanne, is the strongest, most artistic, talented, and incredible person. She lives her life to the fullest, allowing nothing to get in her way. Her determination to take on this project, and the time, creativity, intuitiveness, and sensitivity that she brought to it made what was difficult and emotionally intense genuine and uplifting.

Laurie, outrageous and dynamic, powerful and courageous, is loved and missed. My hope is that her namesake, Luc, inherits her indomitable spirit.

My brother, Greg, who gave me the pep talk of a lifetime, has offered love and support that is immeasurable. My father, Herb, gave me the untiring characteristics of perseverance and determination. Both men have proven that by living with passion one can obtain what they strive for.

A special thank-you to Stephen Scheu. His generosity and comfort was critical. He, along with Dakota and Austin, were an ongoing source of positive energy, never faltering in their love and optimism.

Larry Weinstein, my business partner and true friend, along with my restaurant family, kept my business flourishing. And, I want to thank David's friends at Grey, for being there too.

Ralph Scheu's ground-breaking achievement not only changed our lives, but also set a precedent for all couples so that they do not have to adopt the child that is biologically theirs in the State of Illinois.

I want to thank our support team, each of whom played an invaluable role: Patricia Mendell, Arlene Coustan, Nina Singer, Terry Horwich, Merry Alexander, Hilary Steele, Rosalie and Stephen Luber, and Dr. Leeber Cohen.

From the bottom of my heart I want to thank the entire medical team that was instrumental in the creation of Luc, and to all the pioneers that have advanced the science of in vitro fertilization.

Suzanne, Jennifer, and I want to thank the people at William Morrow: Paul Fedorko, for his vision, and Doris Cooper, our editor, who helped shape this book.

I am lucky to have met Laura Dail, my agent and friend. Her stalwart belief in our story and her shepherding it through a challenging process, was her labor of love.

My incredible husband, David, was always convinced we were meant to be parents. He maintained his focus and determination to make his dream a reality and, together, we made it *our* reality. I thank him for his bravery, support, and love.

Thanks go to our entire famiy for their endless love, and to our dear friends who were compassionate and respectful of our privacy.

Finally thank you to Luc for teaching me the true meaning of life, of happiness and love. You are an incredible baby, a shining star, a special person. You are joyful, loving, charming, delightful, and fun. May you always be this happy. You are greatly loved, you are a miracle and a blessing.

—LIZA WETANSON FREILICHER

My gratitude to all those who were involved in this chapter of my life is immeasurable. To those I have neglected to name, please know that you are in my heart and I thank you for your support.

I'd like to thank my mother for breathing the spirit of life into every day, for giving me the gift of passion, courage, and fortitude.

My children, Dakota and Austin, I thank for their patience, understanding, and willingness to be different. My best friend, Hilary Steele, who is truly my soul mate. A special thanks to my mother's best friend, Merry Alexander, a wonderfully spiritual and gifted healer who has always been so willing to share their stories with me.

My family, Rosalie, Stephen, Jack, and Gabe Luber whose unconditional love has been my safety net.

My stepfather, Stanley Picheny, for being my partner through the agonizing days of my mother's death and sharing his life with us.

A special acknowledgment goes to Arlene Coustan, who threw a lifeline into the "pit" of pain and despair my mother's death left me in and gave me the insight into my own strength.

A heartfelt thank-you to my father-in-law, Ralph Scheu, who not only believed in my choice but changed Illinois state law to allow Liza and David to be declared Luc's parents without adoption proceedings.

To my wonderful caretakers, Christine Couvalaere and Beaula Togara, who nurtured my children and made my world tick.

To Dr. Leeber Cohen and the wonderful nurses at Northwestern Medical faculty foundation whose encouragement and gentle needles helped me through.

To our agent, Laura Dail, who shares our determination and spirit, and our editor, Doris Cooper, for her direction.

To Evalyn Lee who gracefully shared our most private moments with the camera and lent a supportive ear through the last trying trimester.

To my buddies at HRP, Barb, Joan, and Gary, who put up with all my complaints, hormonal moods, and indulgent lunches and worked with me to get back in shape in the months after Luc's birth.

To our writer and my aunt, Suzanne Wetanson, whose intelligent and creative mind put this story on paper, enduring painful memories and long nights. We share the incredible void my mother's absence creates.

To David, who endured the hormones, fears, and moods of two women to bring his biological child into this world. He is truly gifted at sharing his emotions and I thank him for keeping all avenues open during this incredible experience.

To my cousin Liza, my lifelong playmate, we were destined to take care of each other. She always nurtured my various cut knees and injured pride. I thank her for healing my heart and joining our spirits to bring Luc into this world. I have always believed we have the power to make things happen. I thank our mothers for giving us the gift of determination and the unconditional love that binds us.

And to my husband, Stephen, for his unfailing love, support, and commitment. He is the true hero in this story. He believed in my decision and never criticized my motives. Luc's birth has opened my heart again and brought Stephen and me to new depths of our relationship.

—JENNIFER SCHEU

First, I want to acknowledge Luc, for his stout heart and joyous smile. To see him in the arms of his mother as I wrote this book awed me beyond words.

I also want to thank my friend Ed Spielman for his guidance and support.

And a special thanks to Joe Chierchio for his love and patience.

—SUZANNE WETANSON

CONCEIVING LUC

Chapter
1

*L*ooking out the bedroom window of my seventh-floor apartment, I saw only the hazy darkness of an autumnal New York dawn. The garden lights of the Tavern on the Green were out, and when I listened closely, I could hear the beast of New York City making its gentle wake-up growl. In two hours it would roar so loudly I'd have to close the window, but until then I enjoyed the breeze rolling in over the Sheep's Meadow and trees of Central Park.

I escaped from my bed, being careful not to awaken my husband, David, a light sleeper, and tiptoed across our bedroom to the bathroom, where I turned on the shower. When the mirrors began to blur with steam, I stepped under the hot water, flinching as it stung my skin. I scrubbed my body and hair, cleaning the slate in preparation for the new day.

Here, in the shower, I found peace.

"So, anything happening?" Such questions, from friends and family, who meant well but were exasperating, haunted my days. They wanted to know whether David and I had succeeded in becoming pregnant. My gynecologist repeatedly said I was a healthy woman with a healthy reproductive system. There was no reason why I shouldn't conceive. "Relax and enjoy yourself, Liza, keep stress out of your lovemaking," the doctor instructed. But by nature I am obsessive when it comes to accomplishing a task I have determined to undertake, and so, for the last six months I had been using an ovulation kit that the doctor prescribed to determine the most fertile time of my cycle. Every aspect of my life and David's hinged on the report of the ovulation kit. Conception was a high priority that suspended business and social engagements, and it was taking a toll on our tempers.

The warmth and sound of the water eased my body and mind. I knew I had to turn off the faucet, step out, and face the day. I quickly covered myself with the towel, but not before catching my image in the mirror.

The mirror lied. It was begging to tell me I had every right in the world to buy that size-six dress for David's corporate dinner party Saturday night. It was trying to tell me that this brown, curly mass of hair dripping down my back would be coiled into a chic chignon and I would make David proud at the banquet. The mirror lied. People have said I am a Renaissance beauty. Where were they looking? I saw fat and ugly. Thirty-five years old, fat and ugly.

A light from under the bedroom door meant David was awake. He was probably reading the paper, as usual, and waiting for me. He knew it was time. The damned ovulation kit that I practically wore around my neck told him it was time. He asked me, and I told him. When I finished drying off, I opened the bathroom door to the bedroom and got into bed next to my husband. We had intercourse. No foreplay, no romantic music, no erotic conversation. We didn't even turn out the light. I dug my fingernails into my hands, and after an eternity, David was successful. He lay exhausted next to me as I silently counted the minutes, then he got up and took his turn in the solitary haven of the shower. I lay still, afraid to move, except to put a pillow under my hips, imagining it would make progress easier for the tadpolelike sperm I imagined to be valiantly swimming upstream inside of me, an image I believe many women have.

"Coffee, Liza?" David called on his way to the kitchen.

"Thanks." My voice was hollow. He came back with a mug and

handed it to me. It was one routine I had been able to maintain
while the rest of my life was on hold. I sipped the strong, bitter
liquid and watched as David closed the single button on the loosely
constructed gray jacket of his Armani suit. He looked so corporate,
with his impeccable white shirt and the straight knot that held in
place the burgundy foulard tie his mother had sent from Florida for
his last birthday. There were a few "forty-something" gray hairs at
his temples. David looked just like a high-powered advertising executive should. "You must have a wild and vivid fantasy life," I
wanted to tell him, thinking this act we'd just performed could not
have satisfied him. But we never spoke of the sex act. We spoke very
little lately at all and avoided each other. Perhaps what made me
more sad than anything was our loss of touch, of eye contact.

David was going out into the world looking perfect, to his job,
leaving his imperfect wife lying in a mussed bed, terrified to get up
and clean herself lest a fertilized egg be dislodged.

I promised David a child when we were married four years ago. I
never considered that this oath would confront me with such a sense
of obligation. Maybe it was tension or my lack of commitment that
prevented pregnancy. I've heard of that happening. But the fault
couldn't be all mine. Why did I feel I was the one to be judged
wanting? David must share some of the fault. I hated myself and I
hated my husband. For what? For his desire to have a child—an
extension of himself? For being unflinchingly kind and sympathetic
to my fears of childbearing and disgust with the loss of dignity? For
not being able to take all the blame?

With each disappointment our marriage disintegrated further. For
self-protection I tried to look away. But in my heart, I knew that
this scene was another step on the road of a marriage's destruction.
I wondered if David recognized it, too. He looked so perfect. How
could he imagine his life was not?

He kissed my forehead. "Bye. I'll be home after the gym, around
nine." The door clicked as he left.

At last I was alone.

The man who had gotten out of my bed and left the apartment

had become a stranger to me. During sex, David performed as if my body were an inanimate object. There was no flow of mutual desire, no pleasure; it was a job to be done. I missed the David who was my husband, my confidant, my best friend. I stuck my head in the pillow, closed my eyes, and hoped for sleep; then I could dream of my childhood and escape to a time when things were easier and the world seemed smaller and warmer.

I remembered Woodmere Elementary School, the day the big doors opened for the new first graders. Six years old and I still remember how tiny I felt. In particular, I remember that first Christmas recess. The streets of the suburban town were packed with snow. I had been in the house all day with my nose flattened against the frozen windowpane waiting for my cousin Jennifer. Jennifer was the most important person in the world to me—after my mother.

"Finally, she's here!" I burst into the kitchen, where my mother was preparing lunch for Erica, my roly-poly, three-year-old sister. "Jennifer and Aunt Laurie are here," I cried. Mom and I rushed outside to meet them. Jennifer jumped out of the Avanti—we were a car family, all of us, even then—as soon as Aunt Laurie stepped on the brakes. She and I dashed into the house, paying no attention to my other cousin Jack, Jen's brother, and all the toy trucks and trains a two-year-old boy has in tow.

Aunt Laurie was three years my mother's junior, but she seemed like the older sister because she stood a head taller and was protective of her "little" sister. Growing up in a house where both parents worked during the day and went their separate ways in the evening, the sisters had been left unsupervised and became dependent on each other. Laurie was zany and charged ahead like a bull trampling all obstacles. My mother was gentle, conservative, and clever, with equal determination. Aunt Laurie was a large-boned woman. Her features were full: her lips, her nose, her hips, whereas my mother's frame was small, with a doll-like waistline. Some people said the high bridge of her straight nose gave her a haughty look.

I am eight months older than Jennifer, but at that time, when we were six, she was already an inch taller. Jennifer was wearing her dance tutu under her coat. I had already put on mine—with black tights and pink ballet slippers. There was no time to waste.

Jen and I had a mission: we had to prepare a fabulous show for my mother and Aunt Laurie so they would agree to our plea for a weekend sleep-over. We assumed they would be so delighted and proud they would not refuse us. "We'll see" could not be a possible answer. "Yes" is all we would accept.

We dashed off to the den to practice. We felt warm and safe being a part of their world. Safe was important to remember. For me, safe meant being away from large groups, especially strangers. For Jennifer, it was being with her mother. Jen and I, "Princess" and "Lollipop," remained close, like sisters, throughout our childhoods. Just like my mother and Aunt Laurie.

When I was nine years old my father realized his ambition of becoming a self-made millionaire by the age of thirty. He didn't hide his pride or his wealth. We lived in what was truly a castle, brought over to Long Island's south shore from Normandy fifty years before by one of Hewlett Bay Park's settling families. It had passed from that original family and been sold three times, but its authenticity and its integrity had always been maintained. The "castle" was complete with a turret and a suit of armor in the great stone hallway near the fireplace. On the staircase landing was a tapestry with an embroidered coat of arms and a tall Tiffany clock.

On special occasions, my mother would let me spend the weekend at Aunt Laurie's house. It was different up there in Munsey. All the families were of middle income and any failure to keep up with the Joneses was considered a dereliction of duty. I felt no one there liked me, but once I saw Aunt Laurie and Jennifer, I was happy and safe and didn't care what anyone else thought.

We went hiking. Hiking meant exploring streams, jumping from rock to rock, Aunt Laurie in a fabricated sarong that revealed all her full curves, Jennifer, tall as her mother, a cap of bright yellow hair and legs like a stork. I tagged behind, fearful of slipping or stepping on a creature.

Often we would watch Aunt Laurie dance. She was practicing for the lead in the ballet dream sequence of *Oklahoma!* for the community theater group. Aunt Laurie had her own unique interpretive style of dance that was spellbinding. Not just to the audience, but in this case to her costar as well. He found her enchanting, wooed her, put a string of seed pearls around her neck, and gave her a rose at the final curtain. This made her feel as beautiful and as delicate as the pearls. Laurie had been called "big and fat" as a child. At thirteen years old, she had attained her adult height of five feet eleven inches and weighed 180 pounds; she was the target of cruel jokes by her peers—a hurt she couldn't forget, though she eventually shed the extra weight. Laurie loved men. Even after she was married, she couldn't get enough compliments, and bragged about her many admirers to her sister. She enjoyed the power of being able to bestow upon or deny men pleasure. When my aunt entered a room she seemed to fill it: tall and proud, men and women alike couldn't help but stare. She was womanly, with wild curly brown hair and a flaunting attitude.

Of course her marriage to Martin Luber was doomed. They were divorced when Jennifer was ten years old. Laurie stayed in the house with her children and Martin moved to Queens. And though Jennifer missed her father and saw him regularly, she felt her life had not been interrupted by the divorce. In fact, she felt it had become richer because of the mutual dependency that came to exist between her mother and herself. She felt special and she knew she was needed.

Jennifer and I spent many evenings in Aunt Laurie's Victorian bedroom among the downy pillows of antique lace and petit point she prided herself on making. We would watch my aunt parade in front of her mirror slapping her Rubensesque hips as if by will alone she could hammer them away. Because she was dissatisfied with the fit and flow of any store-bought clothing, she would cut up an old dress, drape it, and belt it to camouflage those hips—the bane of her existence. There were scraps of material, threads and pins all over the mauve carpet. In the corner was a mannequin draped in moss-green satin. "Okay, Lollipop, where should we go for dinner tonight?" she asked me, strutting in front of us for our critique on the new creation.

"Let's have pizza. Or Chinese food."

We usually ended up in the kitchen and all pitched in to create a delectable potluck meal.

As much as I enjoyed being with Jennifer and Aunt Laurie, it was my mother who was my true best friend. I confided in her and she was the one who understood my heart. She and I talked together for hours. We talked of my feelings toward boys. I was shy with them, as if they were judgmental of me, and I didn't know how to behave. My girlfriends just treated the boys as pals. I asked my mother if it was because my father didn't pay much attention to me, and she suggested I try a new outlook, to see each person as an individual first and not part of a group. This perspective helped me then and it helps me today not to be intimidated by people. With a warm look or a gentle touch, my mother could reassure me of the strengths we'd discovered in ourselves, and my insecurity would pass. My mother was *home* while my aunt Laurie was *adventure*. With Laurie and Jen, I was a free spirit. With my mother, I was more introspective. As I grew older these two sides of my nature were often at odds, and at times made it difficult for me to make decisions.

Many afternoons my mother and I would sit at my desk and look over my collection of memorabilia. I was a scrupulous hoarder. I saved homework papers with teachers' comments; I had movie stubs on which I'd noted the name of the friend I'd gone out with. We talked about all the bits and pieces and what they meant to me and about the beautiful picture of my life I would have to show my own children. My mother told me how proud she was that she and I shared our intimate thoughts. She confided to me that she was often lonely. I didn't understand loneliness then as I do now. Now, as an adult, I'd think of Jen, living in Chicago with her husband and two children. And of my aunt Laurie. And I felt so alone that it pained me. Where was the child my mother said I would have? My mother was thirty-two years old then, three years younger than I was today, and she had three children.

Where was my child?

·   ·   ·

We were on the patio one summer morning. I was ten years old and just becoming aware of the meaning of adults' conversations. I was understanding that there was more to life than my own circle of pleasures and fears, and what affected my loved ones—my mother— affected me. So I listened and paid attention and thought about what I heard. The sun sparkled on the pool, surrounded by a garden of roses and daisies. My mother brought breakfast out for Grandma Reese. We sat beneath the green-and-white striped awning. I was making designs with my Spirograph kit. Greg and Erica were playing with clay on the floor. My grandmother looked at us, the house and the pool, and said: "Suzy, you are the luckiest girl in the world."

My mother stopped in her tracks and her face drained of color. I knew she was unhappy, despite her apparent blessings: three healthy children, a husband who continually professed his love, and a lavish lifestyle. She didn't say a word and went into the house.

In the midst of paradisical life, I believe my mother had a fore-boding that morning. She was frightened. I followed her into the kitchen and asked her why she had acted so strangely. She gave no explanation and never mentioned what had happened, even during our quiet talks. She kept the premonition to herself, but I know she never forgot my grandmother's words that morning, because years later she told me of the darkness she saw.

At the end of the month, the ache in my back and the cramps in my stomach should have warned me, but when I saw the blood on the sheet in the morning, I started to cry. David was in Cincinnati on business. I was alone and empty inside; there was no baby growing.

I ripped the stained sheets from the bed and replaced them with my favorite periwinkle flowered ones. The window was open wide, filling the room with fresh cool air.

The phone rang. I picked it up knowing it was Jennifer; she always called at this time on her way to work each morning.

"What's the matter?" she said, understanding the tone of my voice so well.

"Stained sheets." It was the quickest, most comprehensive explanation.

"Liza, this has been going on long enough. Don't you think you're burying your head in the sand, not realizing there is a real problem here? It's time for an in-depth physical exam. And a mental one, too, I might add. This isn't like you. Why are you avoiding the reality that there's a reason why you're not pregnant? What are you afraid of? Whatever it is, it can be fixed."

"Jen. I'm late for work," I said, wanting to end this unpleasant conversation.

"Lollipop . . ." she began, drawing me back.

"You're right, Jen. I'll set it up today. Thanks. Bye." I hung up the phone, knowing she was right, knowing I would see the doctor, knowing I was ambivalent. I said I wanted a child and went through the motions of fulfilling David's dream, but something in me was holding me back.

I started Sambuca, the large Manhattan trattoria, when I needed a career. It became my refuge from what I didn't want to deal with. At that time I was too busy to think of a husband or a child. Sambuca was my life and I put all my strength and creativity into it. If I wasn't there, it was my contention; nothing was right. After my marriage it remained the same.

That morning, in the half hour I'd been there, I realized the new party-and-reservations person was not as experienced as she had professed. Despite my high-tech computer program, there was a missing case of wine to account for. When I saw the bartender arranging the glassware unevenly on the shelf, I told him it looked terrible and grabbed his towel and polished and straightened them myself.

"Calm down, Liza, do you want him to quit? You have never spoken to people like that. Tell him nicely, he wants to do a good job."

I hadn't noticed my brother, Greg, come in. He has a restaurant across the street and often stopped by on his rounds to his other five establishments.

The bartender was now taking liquor inventory at the end of the bar. I handed him the towel and apologized. Greg and I went into my office.

"What's up? Something's the matter." His voice was always soft.

At twenty-seven, Greg was not a kid. Although younger, he is tougher and wiser than me in many ways. Happily married, with the most wonderful boy in the world, Stuart, and his wife, Maxine, who was again pregnant, Greg's life was in order. It seemed so easy for him. How could I explain my hurt and disenchantment with my husband? I didn't see our lives going anywhere together.

My brother sat next to me and took my hand. I could see our reflections in the mirror on the opposite wall. The same face, the same thick brown hair. His expression was relaxed, but his dark eyes were full of concern and his strong chin jutted forward proudly. My face was a frown with darting eyes; I looked like a mouse.

I twirled my hair around my fingers. My nervous habit.

"Liza, I haven't seen you like this, jumping all over people. Let go of your hair and tell me what's the matter."

"I got my period this morning."

"Sometimes getting pregnant doesn't happen quickly. Maxine and I were lucky."

"David and I have been trying for six months, taking my temperature, calculating ovulation—"

The phone rang. I reached to answer.

"Let it ring."

I picked it up anyway. "No, we don't serve kosher meals!" I said in a curt voice, and slammed the receiver. "Everything upsets me. I can't concentrate on my business. My employees whisper about me. They think I've become crazy. I don't know what to do. David and I act like cordial roommates, except when we have to have sex. Isn't that awful, to have to have sex and then to wait and hope and be able to think of nothing else?"

Greg took the phone, which was still clenched in my hand. "I always heard you say how ugly pregnant women are and that they must be crazy to put themselves through the pain and lack of dignity. Do you really want that for yourself? Do you want a baby?"

"Of course I want a baby."

"No. No. No. Do you, Liza, want a baby, or are you doing this as a martyr for David? Does Liza want to be a mother?"

"Yes. Yes, I do." My voice, even to my own ears, sounded unconvincing.

"Do you know what it means? Once you become pregnant, that child is what you think of first for the rest of your life. There are moments when I wish I could be alone with just Max. You're the girl who says kids are a pain in the neck. Even Stuart."

"It's not that. I love Stuart. You know how I enjoy being with him." I paused, then admitted, "I'm afraid of the pain of childbirth, and once you are pregnant you have no choice. You can't change your mind. And . . ."

"And? What else?" Greg said. "That's too simple."

Greg saw that getting my period that morning was just a part of what was upsetting me. He knew, unlike anyone else, that there was more to my uneasiness.

"And look at Mommy, what she went through with Erica. How can I take the chance of that happening to my child and me?" Again the phone rang. "A table for six at six o'clock. Yes, we have high chairs. You need two high chairs. We allow strollers—no problem." I clenched my teeth. "Please make sure your party is here together and on time. Thank you." Only because Greg was there did I hang up with composure. Then I burst. "A six-top. Two couples with two kids and two babies in strollers. At the start of dinnertime. They order nothing and the brats drop half of the food on the floor. Would they slop up their own homes like that? No! They order no drinks. I lose money—can't turn the table and all the fucking while the little monsters in the carriages are screaming. The parents are stressed—barely tip the waiter, and leave thinking it's my fault they had a lousy time. Why do people think they must have kids, anyway? I don't know why in the world anyone would want them." I didn't even know I was crying.

Greg turned and faced me straight on. "I'll tell you why," he said. "Because without children, we'd be a hopeless species without purpose. We'd kill each other off and become extinct." The truth was comical. We both laughed. "Liza . . ." His voice became deep and deliberate. "A child's illness is something every parent dreads. But life goes on. You can't stop living because of fear. Erica's illness caused terrible grief, and turmoil for everyone in the family, but let it stop. I can't explain the pure joy Stuart brings me. I can't imagine my life without him. He is my heart and I know my new child will be the same. I am the best, loving, informed parent I can possibly be and that's all I or anyone else can strive for. I hope my children will be happy and well rounded people. Remember what Mommy always says. You have to give to get."

"So what do I do? What can I give?"

"You give total commitment. Make up your mind and go for it. Meanwhile, find out why you haven't conceived."

I kissed him and took the tissue he handed me to wipe my nose. "Thanks. What's wrong with me?"

"Right now it's a mystery. You're a curious girl. Unravel it." He smiled that Greg smile; no one else's mouth forms a perfect square when they smile.

David met me at the restaurant for dinner that evening.

"We have to do something about this problem," I told him. He took a deep breath, glad, at last, to be confronting our difficulty.

"I didn't want to suggest it to you. Neither of us wanted to suspect a problem."

"We can't waste time, David. You're forty-one. I'm thirty-three. Now is the time to start a family. Maybe something is wrong, but there has to be a way to make it happen. The doctor has told me the same thing every six months since we were married. My reproductive system is healthy, I should be able to become pregnant and have a child. He attributes the failure to stress, which he says is common in working women of my age who have conflicting interests. But, David, I'm me, not a member of a group. This time he must tell me why Liza Freilicher has not become pregnant."

∞

I WAITED IMPATIENTLY outside the doctor's examining rooms. I felt insecure about my health. I was the only woman there with a waistline. They were all pregnant, sitting back on the comfortable armchairs, not too deep so they could get out of them with ease. I was so nervous. I could hear my heart pounding in my ears.

I thought back to when Erica was sick. I was nine years old. Her scream awoke me. "Mommy, my head. My head hurts, Mommy."

My mother was in our bedroom before I could get up. She rocked Erica and put cold towels on her forehead. "It's just a bad dream—hush, hush." Then Erica threw up, the vomit spewing across the room. After, she felt better. My mother cleaned her and lulled her to sleep with soft humming and her familiar Brahms lullaby.

In the morning, Erica was well and went cheerfully to kindergarten. "A bad dream." But it happened the next night and the next, until finally my mother took her to Dr. Brenner, our pediatrician. After a week of sleepless nights, of screaming and vomiting, my mother took Erica to Long Island Jewish Hospital.

Dr. Epson, the neurosurgeon, examined her. He looked, searching into her eyes with an opthalmoscope and then asked her to stand with her eyes closed and stretch out her arms. "Now, Erica, touch your pointer finger to the tip of your nose, first with one hand, then the other."

Erica was unable to do this. She touched her ear with one hand and missed her face altogether with the other.

"She has a brain tumor." So quickly he had determined the problem. "There will be many tests to substantiate it, but she has a brain tumor."

That was the day our family and the happy, secure life I'd known began to fall apart. Mother stayed at the hospital day and night. Our life was empty without her. Greg cried daily and crept into my bed at night. He was a baby, two years old, and all of a sudden his mother wasn't there. Finally, my father brought us to her at the hospital for hugs and kisses and promises that she would soon be home. My mother looked tired and stone-faced; it was the expression I had seen before on that hot summer day years ago. The words from long ago echoed in my brain.

Suzy, you are the luckiest girl in the world.

I knew that my childhood was over. That beautiful scene of a healthy carefree family at play was erased and replaced by the blackness my mother had foreseen. I realized that even with forewarning, I was unable to escape life's swift, silent changes. The responsibilities of adulthood replaced the innocence of childhood.

A CAT scan of Erica's head pinpointed a tumor the size of an orange at the base of her brain. It was in an area most doctors considered inoperable. My mother told me she and my father had sat at a large conference table with many doctors and anesthesiologists to decide whether to proceed with the surgery. The chances for success were discussed. The majority were opposed, but Dr. Epson said he believed strongly that he could remove the tumor, though not without great risk. The tumor was growing rapidly and would eventually kill Erica. The ultimate decision was up to my parents. My father turned to my mother, as he always did where we children were concerned. She stood up and looked directly into Dr. Epson's eyes. "Operate," she said in a quiet but definite voice.

Erica stayed in the intensive-care unit for a month, her head wrapped in bandages, her fever rising to 106 degrees and falling well below normal. Mother was there, always. Another mother also waited to see if her little daughter would survive. I watched them both in the waiting room. My mother just looked out the window, imagining herself on the bench under a big tree on the lawn out there. The other woman sat moving her rosary beads methodically through her fingers and mouthing silent prayers. One day the woman wasn't there and the crib in the ICU was empty. My mother told me she never prayed to God after that. She learned not to look elsewhere for strength or miracles, they had to come from within. "You have to make the miracles happen yourself."

Mother nursed Erica for three months in the hospital. She assisted Dr. Epson in painful spinal taps. She draped Erica's frail body in cold towels to bring down her fevers. In the end, Erica recovered, except for the large protrusion of nonabsorbed spinal fluid at the back of her head. Dr. Epson scheduled a shunt—a surgical procedure that would drain the fluid into the heart. Mother had him cancel it, not wanting to put her little daughter at risk again, and took Erica out of the hospital. At home she made Erica swim in the heated pool, twice daily. And one morning, the threatening lump was gone. Flat. The neurosurgeon couldn't believe it. That was my mother's miracle. And it taught me that a person has the ability to persist against all odds and make things happen. This lesson would stay with me forever.

When Erica was better and in school, my mother bolted into the world like a wild animal that had been released from a cage. She rekindled her childhood passion for horseback riding, but this time craved the adrenaline rush that jumping gave her. Her life had been swamped by hospitals and life-and-death decisions. The act of jumping, of overcoming a hurdle was a catharsis.

Many mornings as I was dressing for school she'd run into my room fully dressed in chaps and boots, pull my own gear from the closet, and insist I change and come with her.

"I'd be playing hooky," I said, worried that I would do something wrong.

"Not if you're with your mother," she replied. "Besides," she continued, sensing my hesitation, "you're my daughter and I want to be with you. That's why I had you. Okay?"

"Okay," I said with conviction.

I rode Pal-O-Mine, the biggest horse in the barn. He was docile and I jumped hurdles along with my mother and then we'd have lunch and be home in time for tea in front of the TV, with Greg and Erica watching *Dark Shadows,* our favorite program about vampires.

Aunt Laurie was at our house at least twice a week to visit and see Erica. It was difficult for her to bring Jennifer each time because there was school and someone had to be home for Jack, Jennifer's little brother. One day my aunt gave my mother two skirts she had made. The "belly skirt," as Laurie called it, was cut on a sharp bias and slid over the hip into a gentle fullness. It made my mother look taller than her five feet four inches and she was delighted. The "gypsy skirt" flared in three frivolous tiers from a dropped waist. Aunt Laurie's choice and use of fabric was brilliant; she was making sarongs long before Donna Karan. Mother wore the gypsy skirt whenever she went out. When she and my father went dancing she wore the red belly skirt, which dipped well past her navel, with a red sequined halter. Her naked legs kicked out from the open front when she danced. I called her the "Red Witch." All the men, she told me, admired the outfit, and I know that amused her. But nothing was more exciting than the times when she was flying over fences on her horse, Blacky, early in the morning. That deserved admiration.

Many women wanted the skirts and soon my aunt Laurie was

sewing for the young, affluent Five Towns ladies. The money was a much-needed addition to the paltry child support she and her two children lived on.

"LIZA FREILICHER."

I was jolted from my reverie.

"The doctor will see you."

I glanced out the window. There were no trees, just the overcast sky of New York City. I followed the nurse.

Dr. Silver did a comprehensive examination and gave me a good prognosis for having a child.

"Liza, I know you've been trying to get pregnant. I could tell you it's your age and to see an infertility specialist, but before you do that I think it's a good idea to have your husband's semen examined." He shook my hand. "Don't worry. Everything will be all right."

"All right?" It never occurred to me that the problem could be with David. It was archaic to think it, but in my mind pregnancy and babies were exclusively a woman's realm.

Chapter

3

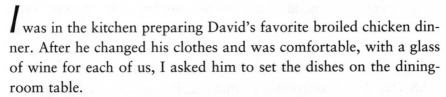

I was in the kitchen preparing David's favorite broiled chicken dinner. After he changed his clothes and was comfortable, with a glass of wine for each of us, I asked him to set the dishes on the dining-room table.

"David, have you ever impregnated a woman?" I called into the dining room. I had waited until he was in the other room so I would not have to see the hurt and vulnerability in his face when I asked.

"Liza? What a question . . . why do you ask?"

"Dr. Silver recommended that you have a semen analysis."

I heard the clink of dishes as David put them on the table. I heard the knives and forks laid down one at a time. "A semen analysis? Then he thinks I could be . . ."

"No. He didn't speculate about anything. He just wants to rule out all possibilities."

"Well, he's right. It takes two people to make a baby. I just never thought . . . I'll make the appointment."

He came into the kitchen and stood in the middle of the room with his arms loose at his sides. "Where?" he asked.

"Mount Sinai."

.　　.　　.

Three days later, on Thursday morning, David went to Mount Sinai for a semen analysis. He was escorted to a closet-sized room with a reclining chair, porno magazines, and videos. It might have been on Forty-second Street, only a little cleaner. "I just wanted to jerk off in a hurry and get out of there," David said later. He felt too awkward and upset to see the humor in the situation . . .

We waited anxiously for the test results, which were to come that evening. We embraced wordlessly during that time. It was strange, I felt closer to David now than I did during our recent lovemaking. It was an intimacy that arose out of need and caring for one another and the understanding that we each suffered for the other. It was a new way of feeling and it strengthened our bond. We kept ourselves closeted in our own world, waiting to hear what seemed like a verdict.

When the call came, David answered. The clinician said, "There is no sperm in your ejaculate."

To us that meant David was sterile. We stood in the kitchen holding each other and sobbing uncontrollably. It meant we'd never have a baby.

I don't remember going to bed that night. I was numb, and when there were no more tears, David and I moved to opposite sides of the bed. During the night, I heard him whimpering. When I looked into his eyes, I saw pain.

When morning came, both David and I believed that if we wanted a child it meant either adopting or opting for donor sperm, a good choice friends had made. David didn't doubt his masculinity when he learned he might be sterile, it was that he felt cheated. He wanted his biological child. He felt entitled to it. Most people can naturally produce a child, an extension of themselves. Why not us? To David, getting married meant having a family and raising his own child.

For me the question of donor sperm was frightening. Like adoption, it was opening the door to the unknown. What was the genetic background of the donor? What were the inherent risks of illness or negative personality traits? We would never be able to look at our child and say "He looks like you."

After the results of the semen tests were confirmed, David's urologist at Mount Sinai gave us the name of an infertility psychologist.

He assured David that she was very informed and would be able to educate us about our various alternatives to get a baby.

We consulted Patricia Greene in her downtown office. In her late forties, Patricia was a woman with an infectiously bright outlook. She spoke frankly, without mincing words. On the day we met, she was dressed casually in a navy-blue mid-calf skirt and ivory sweater. Fresh daisies graced her office. There were no family pictures on her desk and the paintings that decorated the walls were abstract and impersonal. I never learned about Patricia's private life. She seemed to avoid any personal questions. Perhaps, I thought I would find a friend in the psychologist or a big sister, but that couldn't be, I realized, if she were to be objective. Once I understood the strictly professional nature of our relationship, Patricia became my sounding board, the person to whom I could confess my anger and get to its source. I had created a picture in my mind of my relationship with David that was not completely the truth. Patricia didn't make judgments but listened and gave information and advice only after she had reached an understanding of each of us as individuals and as a couple. David and I felt confident that Patricia had seen us as unique individuals and not put us in a predetermined category, which, I was afraid, was the practice of many psychologists.

It was somewhat comforting to David and to me to learn that 18 to 20 percent of couples suffer from infertility. All too often infertility is looked upon as something shameful, rather than as a circumstance that can be dealt with. Patricia made it clear to us that if David were sterile our options were donor sperm or adoption. Both choices were troubling, but she helped us realize that they were the only ways for us to have a child.

With Patricia's guidance, we decided on donor sperm. The child would at least come from my body. I was adamant about this. I didn't want to bring up a child without some biological connection to me or my husband. I wanted my baby from my egg, with genes from my body.

We were also warned that if we decided never to tell the baby that David was not its genetic father this secret must not be told to anyone, ever. Not even to my own mother.

This was very upsetting to me. I don't believe in secrets. I never had secrets from my mother, Greg, or Jennifer. How could I keep my child's lineage hidden from him? How could I found a child's whole life on a lie?

"Liza," David said as we left Patricia's downtown office, "let's keep quiet for now. We can reserve the right to decide later."

I agreed not to cause him more anguish, knowing that if I chose donor insemination and became pregnant, I would insist we tell our child the truth, and make him understand that genetics has nothing to do with love.

The next step was to research the many sperm banks. We were sent piles of profiles. It seemed impossible to commit to one. We agreed that the donor should be Jewish, as we were. Should he have brown eyes like mine, blue like David's? We insisted that the baby have the proper blood type so when he had a blood test it wouldn't raise any question about who his parents were.

David's priority was brains.

After the terrible experience of hospitals and illness in my family, my concern was health and longevity.

When the profiles arrived we went into separate rooms so as not to influence each other. We each marked the possibilities we liked, then we compared notes. We did this for weeks and weeks. Both David and I felt awkward. It was like going shopping. Finally we made a selection, a donor who had everything: Jewish, blue eyes like David, a little short, from a family of college graduates and aged grandparents.

There was no excitement. There was, for me, a sense of unreality. I never was a gambler. I felt as if we were putting all our hopes on a number on a roulette wheel. This sperm would fuse with the life essence of my body and produce a child.

David was brave and told me that with my egg it was still his son; his name and future were secure. I couldn't imagine this sacrifice, yet David accepted the situation and was willing to commit himself fully. So badly did he want a child.

The sperm bank manager said straight-faced and confidently, "Oh, number 2047. I've seen his offspring; they're beautiful. Everyone wants him; he's our most popular." We bought his sperm. We even bought extra inventory of #2047 in case later on we wanted another sibling with the same genetic makeup. We rented a nitrogen-oxide tank to hold the sperm and had it messengered to the infertility clinic at Mount Sinai Hospital in New York.

Before I made the appointment for insemination by #2047, David wanted to see another urologist at Mount Sinai and have a final semen analysis and opinion. "Laboratories make mistakes and doctors are human and there may be another option—surgery or medication, even diet or exercise," he said, hoping against hope.

Again the test proved he was aspermatic. But this time the doctor suggested a testicular biopsy to see if there were any sperm impacted.

I found it annoying and infuriating that this possibility had not been suggested in the first place. It would have saved me and David a lot of pain, not to mention all the time wasted on chosing a sperm donor. Cautiously, we pushed to schedule the biopsy within the week.

The procedure proved that David had viable sperm.

This was exciting news. We had our dream back. But as it turned out, David's sperm could not be extracted because it was too immature to fertilize an egg. The solution for us to get pregnant naturally would be reconstructive surgery in the hope that the sperm would be able to mature as it completed its journey through the vas deferens.

The doctors believed that the obstruction was caused by scar tissue. As a teenager, David had had a urological infection accompanied by a high fever that lasted for three days. This could have caused the scarring.

David went for the surgery as he had gone to work each morning. He was dressed for business. His face was firm. He was the image of confidence. His goal was in sight—his baby. If surgery was one of the stops along the way, so be it.

As we entered the hospital, the smell, the hushed, busy impersonal atmosphere awakened all my old fears of doctors. David squeezed my hand as he was taken to the operating room. "We'll be fine," he said, to bolster my courage. I should have been the strong one for him; instead, I found myself a quivering child. I was disgusted with myself.

Instead of the expected two hours, David was on the table for five.

"Why is it taking so long?" I asked the nurse each time she came into the waiting room where I was pacing.

"He's doing well" is all she said after I had her call down to the OR for the sixth time.

I feared the doctor had changed his prognosis and David's condition was not reversible. We wanted this cure so badly. If the surgery was successful, David would be ejaculating sperm and we'd have a good chance for pregnancy. In David's mind, he had no choice. He felt it was his problem and he would do anything necessary to be our child's biological father.

Finally the doctor stepped into the waiting room.

"Sit down, Liza. Your husband is fine, he's in the recovery room. You can see him shortly. David does have sperm, but I was unable to repair the blockage. After he has healed, I will be able to surgically extract sperm."

I was shaking and sweating and freezing, "What does that mean? I thought the sperm was too immature to be able to fertilize my eggs?"

"That is true," the doctor said. "You will have to go through in vitro fertilization and then David's sperm can be injected into the harvested egg through a process called intracytoplasmic sperm injection, or ICSI. Do you know about this type of assisted reproductive technology?"

"No," I said, still devastated by the failure of the surgery.

"In vitro fertilization—(IVF)—is an assisted pregnancy. A woman is given a cycle of hormones to stimulate the ovaries to produce more than one mature egg. When the eggs are ripe, another hormone is administered to cause the follicles in the fallopian tubes to release the eggs into the uterus. The ripe eggs are then retrieved from the uterus and placed in a glass culture dish with sperm, where they become fertilized. If the sperm is immature and not viable, they are injected into the egg by an embryologist. This process of injecting the sperm directly into the egg is called ICSI, introcytoplasmic sperm injection. After fertilization it is determined how many of the fertilized eggs, now called embryos, will be transferred to the uterus. If an embryo adheres to the uterine wall and cell division continues, pregnancy is achieved and goes ahead naturally.

"The infertility clinic here at the hospital has an advanced program," David's urologist continued. "Call the counselors there. They will explain and get you started."

Chapter

4

Now we had another option, IVF, or fertilization outside the body, in a small glass circular disk, in a laboratory. That was the next step if we wanted our biological child. It was early spring '95. We went to the infertility clinic at Mount Sinai. I sat and listened to the procedure of drug administration, egg development, and retrieval that in vitro entailed. In vitro would cause me to produce multiple eggs. They would ripen and be retrieved in the hospital vaginally, using a special catheter.

At the time my eggs would be retrieved, David's sperm would be aspirated and brought into the laboratory. My eggs would then be fertilized with his sperm. A single sperm would be injected, by the embryologist, directly into each retrieved ripe egg. After fertilization and cell division, the embryo would be implanted, vaginally, into my uterus.

As the counselor spoke, it seemed unbelievable to me that her words pertained to David and me. I, of all people, who mistrusted doctors and became teary each time I went near a hospital. I, who trembles at the sight of a needle. Yet the technical explanation made sense. I weighed the relief of knowing I could possibly have a child against the horror this new procedure aroused in me, and couldn't give myself an honest answer how I would decide. Did I have the strength and dedication to follow through? I honestly didn't know.

IVF, I was told at the clinic, has numerous risks and is therefore controversial. The risks from the medications were not completely known, but included ovarian cancer and hyperstimulation of the ovaries.

David and I spent months researching the procedure and checking out institutions around the country where it was performed. Suddenly I found that in vitro was being pursued by almost all the women I knew who were hoping for a baby. My neighbor Hanna, who, after three attempts, was pregnant with twins; Allison, the daughter-in-law of my mother's friend, was pregnant after her first cycle; and my friend Mindy was on her sixth attempt. In vitro seemed to have a strange effect on women. To most it was an ugly secret they kept concealed; others became addictive to it; they refused to give up.

To me it became an obsession. I needed to learn all I could about IVF. Knowledge helped me feel that I had some sense of control.

⁂

DAVID AND I HAVE a house in Watermill, Long Island. It is a two-hour drive from New York City, but once you are there you are in a sublime place that hugs both ocean and farmland. This was our haven. Our house borders on a cornfield with an old red barn. The sunsets during those spring and summer months of 1995 were incredibly beautiful—that fiery ball sinking behind the cornstalks, with wild geese flying overhead. Four months had passed since David's surgery. We had chosen to begin IVF, and although I was terrified of the drugs, the injections, the surgeries, the doctors, and losing my dignity, here at the house I was at peace with the hope of having a biological child. Here, away from doctors and hospitals, seeing gardens and birds and nature's constant rebirth, I felt sure this was the right decision.

We had been working together toward one goal without inwardly blaming each other. We had been communicative. David , from time to time, looked at me like a man who desires his mate. Yet, during his healing, we had not made love.

At the house, during this hiatus, I tried to put thoughts of IVF out of my head. I refinished my garden furniture and a bench for the front hall. I plastered the walls in the living room. I planted a walled perennial flower garden with roses and hollyhocks that threatened to obliterate the path to my front door. Just being outside in the air made me happy. The sun felt wonderful, warming my back.

In the fall, when we went back to the clinic, we were as informed on the subject of IVF as the doctors themselves. When asked at the infertility clinic if we were both totally committed as a couple, David and I said yes and signed the consent form, but deep inside I knew my ambivalence about having a baby was still strong. Back again in the world of doctors and hospitals, all that I dreaded returned to the surface, and though I signed the commitment form, I was confused and terrified. The IVF process would begin. Some days I would receive up to five injections. There would be daily blood tests and then repeated sonograms to watch my egg development.

I resented these procedures. If the choice of in vitro didn't exist, then there would be no drugs. I would choose the donor-sperm method. I wouldn't have to have my eggs harvested, to be inseminated by ICSI. With donor sperm, my eggs would have been artificially inseminated vaginally at the natural time of ovulation.

I dreaded the injections that came with IVF, and what the hormones would do to me. I hated the fact that David had to go through surgery. My mother was no consolation. She was against my injecting drugs into my body.

"Adopt," she said. "It will be your baby. You'll care for an adopted baby and love it. That baby will be your own."

"In all fairness to myself and to David, how can I adopt a child when I know I could possibly have our own biological child? How selfish that would be. It's a wicked trade-off."

"Liza, those drugs are risky. No one knows the long-term results. I don't want you being a guinea pig," my mother argued.

"I don't understand. With Erica you were determined no matter what the odds. Why is it different with me?"

"Because this is not a life-or-death matter. You don't have to jeopardize yourself and take medicine that, who knows in what way, may harm you. You have a choice, Liza. It's a happy choice. One way or another—adoption or donor sperm, you'll have a baby. I don't want to take chances with you. After all, you are my child. You know what you have now, don't make a decision that may open the door for trouble. Disaster happens in an instant."

MOTHER'S DAY, 1972, dawned clear and warm, a sharp contrast to the heavy rain that howled outside our window during the night. Mommy was looking forward to her riding lessons that morning. There was an indoor riding arena at Flying Horse Farms, and come rain or shine, it was her day. She wanted to go. Daddy also was taking a lesson to please her. It was out of character for him; I suppose my mother told him how lonely she was and warned that if he didn't share some of her interests and start recognizing her as a person, someone else soon would. Mother had brought him a riding habit and he looked very handsome. After an early breakfast we set out as a family to Muttontown—my parents, Erica, Greg, and me.

An hour later we were on the North Shore of eastern Long Island. The brown dome of the barn was visible above the trees. I had been to Flying Horse Farms many times with my mother and played with a few kids who were also watching their parents ride. I enjoyed being there. Old Firefly, Joachim Stryker's legendary Olympic jumping horse, was out at pasture. All of us kids loved the big red horse. What a hypnotizing story that was, of how this ungainly plow horse, ready for the glue factory, jumped out of any corral he was put into. Fences couldn't contain him. Joachim Stryker, an immigrant from Belgium, had a long history, for his young years, as a horse trainer and competitive rider throughout Europe. He recognized in Firefly a talent never seen in the most selectively bred jumper, and an opportunity to make his mark in America. He scraped a few dollars together and bought the "worthless animal," schooled him, competed in, and won many equestrian championships.

Firefly and Joachim Stryker, together, earned the money that bought Flying Horse Farms. Firefly deserved his own corral.

Joachim Stryker became an esteemed horse trainer and equitation coach. He traveled the horse show circuit and appeared at Madison Square Garden with Firefly. This earned him the elite title of "Head of the East Island Hunt." That, no doubt, was part of the reason why boarding a horse at Flying Horse Farms was a costly privilege.

We parked alongside the large indoor arena. Already a number of riders were working their horses. I stood in the doorway to watch while my mother pulled her saddle from the car. Sawdust flew up from the horses' hooves and churned in the large space, creating a mist through which the horses moved. I loved the smell of warm hay, sawdust, and the sweating horses.

Joachim Stryker met us at the entrance to the big barn. He was a short man, prone to casting his eyes downward, and was wearing a brown hat and mud-splattered boots. "Good morning," my mother greeted him as she brought her horse, Blacky, out into the sunlight. "Are we having the lesson indoors today?"

Mr. Stryker had been in this country long enough to get married and put three children through high school, but he still spoke imperfect English. "You want to learn to ride? You ride in all weather. We have it outside."

"I'm surprised. It rained so hard last night."

He glared at her. How dare anyone question him? "Sue-Sue, you want to ride in the hunt, you ride in all weather," he repeated, and disappeared into the barn. My mother, only wanting his approval, mounted Blacky and walked down the hill to the hunt course that was set up in the field below. My father came out of the barn mounted on a brown horse. I led Erica and Greg down onto the field after them. Our feet made squishing sounds in the mud.

Mother put Blacky through all the gaits to warm up for the lesson. She posted gently to the trot as Blacky was led in figure eight patterns, changing leads at each loop. She pressed him into a canter

and sat back in the saddle. Then she moved forward, her weight on
her knees in the jump position. I turned and saw Mr. Stryker standing by the imposing pile of stacked tree trunks, the final jump at the
hunt course. The lesson had begun.

Mother did the first run slowly but well. The two-in-one, the in-
and-out; I knew the names. Now it was my father's turn. Mr. Stryker
lowered the rails and Daddy jumped the beginner fences. He looked
pleased with himself. Greg and Erica were poking in puddles by their
feet with sticks. Then it was Mommy's turn again. Mr. Stryker raised
the rails and moved over to the broad obstacle of tree trunks.

"That's it," he called as she crossed each fence without a fault;
no touch, no knockdown.

It appeared my mother had gained confidence. She and Blacky
crossed the barriers without a hitch. As she galloped toward the last
hurdle, Blacky was given the signal and gathered himself for the
jump.

Erica and Greg were throwing stones into the puddle at our feet.

"Greg—no splashing!" I grabbed the stone from his hand and
looked up to see the horse rise and cross the log barrier. Then, in
an instant, I saw him slip as his front hooves hit the wet turf. He
fell to the side, and my mother, still in the saddle, went down with
him. Blacky struggled to his feet and galloped away. My mother lay
motionless. Daddy ran to her, but still she did not move.

"Get up, Mommy," I prayed, putting my arm around Erica to
stop her from running forward. I sensed I had to keep my baby
brother and sister from the sight. It seemed a long time and then I
heard a siren, an ugly, urgent noise. An ambulance drove down the
hill onto the field. Then I saw, through the crowd, my mother's still
body being lifted onto a stretcher.

The paramedics heaved the stretcher into the ambulance and sped
away in a blur of lights and sirens, with my mother, father, and my
whole life inside it.

Erica, Greg, and I were alone. Something terrible had happened,
I knew that. We were taken into the office, given cookies, I think,
and told to wait. My aunt Ilene, Daddy's younger sister, eventually
came and took us home.

I felt like a bomb was about to go off. No one would tell me anything. In fact, no one ever told me, but eventually, from listening to whispers and seeing the distraught faces of my grandmothers, I knew that my mother wasn't coming home for a long while, that she was in the hospital with my father, that she had hurt her back. And I knew from the way my mother looked lying on the ground that she would never, never walk again.

I was eleven years old. I didn't know what a pivotal time in my life this was. My homelife, my family, health, and well-being, these things that I cherished yet took for granted, were abruptly demolished. Once again, hospitals and illness separated our family.

A week went by. I refused to go to school. My father and Aunt Laurie were at the hospital. My grandmothers moved as if in a fog. Our housekeeper, Dora, who had cared for all of us since Greg was born, took over the household. She was busy answering the telephone inquiries of neighbors and friends, shopping, cooking. Two days later my mother was moved by ambulance to New York University Hospital. Dr. Randolf, a renowned neurosurgeon specializing in spinal surgery, was there. He repaired the broken vertebrae and fused them, but he was unable to repair the damage to the nerves of the spinal cord. My mother would not walk again. I knew this before the doctors told me because Dora and Aunt Ilene kept us close and offered us whatever they thought we wanted—ice cream, toys, attention. All I wanted was my mother.

The next week Aunt Laurie came to take me home with her. She let Jennifer miss school, hoping we would play. But all I wanted was to go to New York to see my mother, and so she brought me to the hospital.

Jennifer waited outside Mommy's room while Daddy took me in to her. I was scared. I didn't want to see my mother in pain. "Mommy, please get up." I whispered a prayer, as panic overwhelmed me. I begged God to let me wake up and make this be a dream. I promised never to do anything wrong. Was I being punished for playing hooky? What did I do? What did Mommy do? My thoughts and prayers and fury collided. I didn't understand my new place in life. I tried to control my sobs. *Suzy, you are the luckiest girl in the world.* Why had my grandmother said that? Had she called attention to all we had only to have it snatched away?

My mother was lying still, with tubes attached to her arms. Tears fell over the black-and-blue bruises of her face and made the swollen, stretched skin shine. She tried to talk. I could tell she wanted to say, "La La, I love you," but all she did was turn her face away and reach for my hand. Her touch was so weak.

After a while my father walked me to the hallway, where Jennifer was waiting. Her face was tearstained and she held her mother's hand tightly, afraid that they, too, might be separated. Aunt Laurie took me with her other hand and the three of us sat in the waiting room quietly gazing at the East River with its slow moving barges.

My father and I drove home together. We didn't talk. He couldn't answer my questions. He, too, was separated from the one person who gave him warmth and security. He was needing his wife, although I did not realize it at the time.

After two months my mother was transferred, in a wheelchair, to Rusk Institute at NYU for rehabilitation. She kept her eyes in her book, *The Call of the Wild*. It was a story of devotion and stamina and it took her far away from her surroundings. She spoke to no one in the therapy room, feeling that to accept the help they offered was to concede to being dependent. She refused to cooperate. She had not changed since the accident; she was the same independent woman, with a life of her own, children who needed her, and a husband waiting for her to come home and resume life. She would find her own way, the way she had done when Erica was sick. She didn't need anyone—until she met Leo Perez. He was working as an aide in the therapy room, bringing towels and weights to patients or moving them from wheelchair to the exercise platform.

In Ecuador, Leo had been a CPA. He came to America to make a new life and send for his mother and young son. Leo was a gentle man, thirty-three years old, the same age as my mother. He had heard the therapist say that she would never walk and had looked at her chart. He had seen the fierce look in her eyes when she'd see patients wearing braces and moving between the parallel bars. He recognized her determination, and its source in courage and anger.

He came to her one day. "Excuse me," he said in broken English. "I can make you walk, if you help me."

She looked up at him from her chair with surprise. No one had given her hope of ever being able to do more than sit erect. No doctor had said she might stand up except strapped to a tilt table.

"It will be hard work. Will you do it?"

"Yes," she said.

Years later, the infertility doctor would put the same proposal to me. "In vitro is hard work. Will you do it?"

"Yes," I said, with the same determination my mother had felt when she answered Leo. "Yes." Then I signed the consent form for IVF with my husband.

Mother let Leo move her to the mat and they began to work her arms with light weights.

At the end of the day, Leo would come to my mother's room. He spoke little English, but she had studied Spanish in school. He helped her with Spanish and she taught him English. Leo told my mother he would help her walk with braces. She accepted his challenge and worked hard with him in the therapy room.

At the end of the summer, Mother left the hospital in time to celebrate her birthday at home. She was given a wheelchair, a sheepish smile, and a wave by the therapists. Leo left the hospital also. My father gave him a job in the accounting department of his company. Each afternoon he came to our house and worked with Mother on the parallel bars. She wore heavy leg braces and a metal corset that was strapped up to her armpits. Mother and Leo worked in the bedroom behind closed doors. I could hear her dragging herself or flinging down the crutches, falling into Leo's arms and cursing at him. He paid no attention, was patient yet persistent and encouraging. "You will do it," he said. Then they worked again and again—longer each day. No one expected my mother ever to be erect. Yet the time came when she and Leo ordered plastic leg braces. Lightweight and molded to her legs, they could be worn invisibly beneath her skirts. They were the most beautiful things my mother had ever seen. Leo began to take her out in the day—without a wheelchair. She was able to move gracefully with a walker. They'd go to the grocery store to buy vegetables or to school to see me or Erica in a play, or to help the teacher in Greg's nursery school introduce the children to the thrill of color through finger painting.

· · ·

Exactly what Leo's position was in our lives was confusing to me. In many ways, he played a fatherly role. He took us on outings, to amusement parks, or fishing. We all played ball and swam together—the things I expected my father to do.

We had no family life. My father was always working and rarely came home. My mother went to sleep early, tired from the day's exercise and, I believe, trying to avoid my father and the discontent she saw in his eyes. I spent every night after dinner in my room feeling lonesome and at sea in the world.

I had become sexually aware over the course of the year since my mother's injury. I envisioned my sexuality as a physical entity made up of three parts—like a snowman. The smallest ball, on the top, was free-spirited and pleasure seeking. In the movies, people like that are portrayed as floozies, but they seemed happy and I wouldn't call them bad. Men of this ilk were called romantic names like Don Juan and looked dashing.

The ball in the middle was violence and invasion. Although I knew about rape and submission, I wasn't fearful. I was cautious around strange men, but I never thought I was in danger. I was struck, however, by the violence of childbirth, the hard labor, the blood, and the screams I'd read about and seen in animals. When I thought of childbirth, I was scared.

The largest part of the snowman, on the bottom, was morality— pride, shame, and guilt. This was where my confusion lay. I didn't believe my body or sex was shameful. No one ever suggested or taught me anything of the sort. I believed that my mother had had only one sexual partner—my father, yet often I wondered if she and Leo had been lovers behind the bedroom door. Even though I wasn't afraid to talk to my mother about anything, I didn't, until recently, ask her if she and Leo had been lovers.

She said no, they hadn't. I was disappointed, and saddened. I would have liked to think that she and Leo had had their own beautiful memories to treasure.

For me, during the years when Leo was teaching my mother to walk again, sex was an enigma. I couldn't make the connection between the beauteous joy of lovemaking and the brutality of childbirth. In my many conversations with Jennifer, I learned that she saw childbirth quite differently.

She told me, "Giving birth is a natural function of a woman's body, comforting as a heartbeat and as necessary for the continuance of life. Life is strong and its creation must be powerful like that of the earth. Don't recoil from it, Liza, embrace it and it won't hurt you."

Jennifer's greatest moments were the birth of her two children, Dakota and Austin.

My mother's reentry into life came when she decided to say, "No is not an option." She wouldn't accept anything less. I listened to Jennifer's words and evaluated my desires to have a child and I knew "no" would not be an option for me either. I was powerful. I would have my own biological child—mine and David's. David and I signed the IVF commitment papers.

Chapter

5

Now that I was pursuing in vitro with the firm hope of having a child, I considered my responsibility as a mother. Until then my thoughts had never gone further than the act of giving birth. I hadn't thought of myself as a mother. I reflected on the loneliness of my teenage years and wondered if it was possible to protect my child from that pain. I thought of my mother's anguish during Erica's illness and of the fragility of happiness. I thought of all my encounters with children and in what way they had affected my life.

SUPERSTITION SAYS THAT bad luck runs in series of three. For my family it was true. For ten years, my father had been the hamburger king of the East Coast, owning and operating seventy fast-food restaurants in New York, New Jersey, and Connecticut. However, when McDonald's and Burger King came on the scene, and flooded the radio and television with their ads, kids would settle for nothing but Ronald McDonald. It turned his business around; he was forced to sell.

I was a freshman in high school at that time. My life had changed so much since my mother's accident that I no longer felt a connection with my friends in school. But I found no purpose in staying home either. I got a job after school selling shoes at Jildor, a busy high-style shop in Cedarhurst, the town next to ours. Usually I walked or took the bus to work. Sometimes my mother would surprise me and give me a lift. Leo had taught her to drive with hand controls, and I was so happy to see her waiting for me outside the school gates.

Although on the surface we seemed well off, the family was struggling. Our big house had no heat because we were so deeply in debt that none of the oil companies would deliver to us. Still as unbelievable as it sounds, that summer our family packed up and went, for the first time, to Spain. Ironically, we were able to do this because renting our house on Long Island made more financial sense than living in it.

In September 1976, Aunt Laurie moved to Hewlett. She wanted to be close to her sister and to the clients for whom she sewed her exquisite garments. Jennifer was excited to begin her sophomore year in the same grade and high school as me. She thought we would again be "Princess" and "Lollipop" together, with the rest of the school crowd orbiting around us. As things turned out, though, we weren't the bosom buddies of yesteryear.

I felt obligated to be with my mother; she was alone every day except when she worked with Leo. Many of her longtime friends had disappeared, not wanting to see their own vulnerability reflected in her face. I worked at a shoe store, or I stayed in my room where it calmed me to organize my books and papers and do my homework.

Jennifer loved me, and in her eyes I was the most popular girl in the sophomore class. She was wrong. I had no school spirit. I paid no attention to the "in" crowd, to how they interacted, or cared about whom they gossiped. I attended my classes, went to work, and came home. I know Jennifer depended on me to win her entrée into the crowd, but that wasn't part of my life. I knew then that I was disappointing her. It wasn't intentional. I didn't have the time or the interest and Jennifer took it personally. She was hurt, and felt she didn't fit in at a time in life when fitting in can be crucial.

But there was more to my behavior than just my apathy.

Jennifer said, "Liza, you live in a mansion and have rich friends. I live in the garden apartments. My mother sews for their mothers."

I was so absorbed in my own life that I didn't pay attention to her words. Financial status was coming between us.

She was the prettiest girl in school—long legs, blond hair, and wide green eyes, and the boys pursued her. She had the body of a bombshell and the face of an angel. This made the girls jealous and they snubbed her completely. She wasn't invited to parties. They were mean, and I didn't notice. Jennifer was unhappy and alone.

Jennifer's brother, Jack, was also causing trouble at home. Since Aunt Laurie's divorce, he had become headstrong and unruly. Jack failed school and became impossible to handle. Mother didn't like him coming to our house either and refused to watch him for Aunt Laurie. He was an instigator and would bully Greg into climbing tall trees or taking baseballs from bigger boys, usually resulting in a bloody nose and always in tears. My mother and Laurie were at odds. So were Jennifer and I. No one was happy.

Jack was sent to boarding school at the age of eleven. Laurie and Jennifer lived alone in the apartment together, the way Jennifer had always hoped.

But her contentment was short-lived. Along came Miles Linder, who had been in love with Laurie since their school days. He didn't charm her then and he couldn't do it now. He was a Milquetoast of a man, but now he was a wealthy Milquetoast. Without much encouragement, Miles left his family and took an apartment in New York City for himself, Laurie, and Jennifer. The timing was right. Jennifer and I were on the outs and Laurie was ready to expand her business to the fashion boutiques of Greenwich Village, SoHo, and the Upper East Side. Nonetheless, Jennifer's need for her mother was unchanged and Miles was horning in on her territory. She didn't want to share her mother's attention with him. She began to prance around the apartment in her bra and bikini panties, anything to distract Miles from her mother.

Jennifer and Laurie were constantly arguing. Jennifer accused her mother of allowing Miles to interfere with their relationship, and felt that Miles and her mother's sewing career had pushed her to secondary status.

Laurie argued that Jennifer was embarrassing her, making a spectacle of herself.

One day Jennifer was standing in the center of the room surrounded by bolts of fabric and spools of thread, her hands on her hips, speaking loudly over the constant whir of the sewing machine. "How can you have time for me when he's always around or wanting to go out? I'm the one who's alone. I wish he weren't here and we could be together like before. You don't love him."

"No. I don't," Laurie said honestly, looking up from her work. "I thought having a man around would make a better family structure for you and Jack. I thought Jack could come home from school. You talk about Liza's family as if you were missing a father figure in your life. I wanted to give you one. Children need both parents."

"I just need you," Jennifer said, and stormed out of the room.

Eventually, Laurie grew tired of Miles. She had accumulated a nice-sized bank account of her own, and realized her plan for a two-parent family had been a fantasy. Out Miles went. They had been together for eight months. It was a victory for Jennifer.

After Jennifer and Aunt Laurie moved to New York City, our lives drifted apart. I started dating Richie Olan, the first boy to crack my shell of solitude. Richie and I had a group of friends with whom we double-dated. When we were in twelfth grade, we drove into Manhattan to go to Xenon and Studio 54. Since Jennifer frequented such discos, I often saw her and her girlfriends across the smoke-filled dance floor. There was Jennifer up against the speaker, bumping and grinding to the rhythm, her long blond hair flying wildly. She was virtually naked except for a black tulle sarong sash around her hips and a mini cropped T-shirt, the strobe lights playing dizzying patterns on her sweat-glistening body. I was embarrassed for her. Usually I pretended I didn't see her, and if we actually came face-to-face, I'd say hi and continue on.

Aunt Laurie was living with another man.

I heard that Jennifer had taken up with a spiffy Italian guy in the beauty-parlor business. There were also rumors that he was a heavy gambler and drinker. Aunt Laurie was very upset. Jennifer moved out to New Jersey with him. Her image grew worse. Jennifer now calls this time her "leather period": she sported tight black leather dresses, black lace stockings, and spike heels. Her hair was frosted, teased, and sprayed into a "do."

Today she doesn't like to be reminded of this time in her life. She says it was her way of punishing her mother. Seeing the heartache parents and children can bring to each other, I again realized the tremendous diligence it takes to be a mother, and questioned my willingness.

In the spring, before graduation, we sold our house, this fortress that had been my home. Everything was to be ticketed and sold. I helped my mother and Dora tag and place the Limoges china and silver service on the long mahogany table. The crystal wineglasses and oversized banquet cloths, all treasured things I thought would be in my own home one day were ticketed. We needed the money, true, but those possessions of my mother's? Even the priceless Tiffany clock was sold to a private collector. On sale day, the lines formed at seven A.M. and the traffic continued until dark, when I closed the front door. All those prying eyes looking in our closets, greedy hands opening the drawers to the furniture we had put our clean clothes in; it was an invasion. By the end of the weekend, it was a clean sweep of my childhood.

I enrolled at American University in Washington, D.C. My father paid my tuition and insisted I work to support myself. Carefree college life was alien to me. I had no interest in dating or in my studies. I wanted to prove my worth to my father. I strove to realize someone else's expectations; I stopped trying to know myself. Later, as I contemplated in vitro and having my own child, I wondered if I was clinging to the idea of a childhood I should have had but didn't have.

Jennifer left the world of blow-dryers and hair dye and followed me to American University. She could have gone to any school, but chose American University because I was there.

I in no way prompted her decision and was quite surprised when she told me, with enthusiasm, that she would be my classmate. Today, when we talk about it, and we reminisce together often, she confesses, "I always wanted to live and be like you, La La: doing what was expected of me, having the right friends, the right address, the right school, not moving from house to house, having a family with no invading strangers. My lifestyle was outrageous, a whirl-wind. Yours was sober."

"Jen, you never saw the truth. I was busy working because I was miserable. I wasn't the popular, self-sufficient rah-rah coed you thought I was. You saw what you wanted to see, that's why I hurt you."

"You were my ideal."

"Don't think of me as a fraud. I didn't try to hide from you. I was hiding from myself. Do you love me less?"

"No, no. I love you more, for your honesty and knowing we both are fighting to overcome a hurtful emptiness."

IN THE SUMMER of 1982 my mother and father separated. Again we were spending the summer on the Costa del Sol in Spain, and that June I found love for the first time. His name was Rafael Bartos. He worked for a real-estate firm in Spain. He was slim, of medium height, with sun-darkened skin and sharp, irregular features, but it was his eyes that told you he was Spanish to the core. They were deep and sultry and looked directly into mine. He had no interest in learning English. He was a private, self-confident man, a man eighteen years older than I was, who had custody of his two sons, Adolfo, nine, and Juan, six. They were well-mannered boys. Rafael gave me solace and serenity. His life was orderly. We spent time walking and talking together about our philosophies of life. He didn't look for outside entertainment. Our being together was all he wanted. He was happy seeing me with his boys. We spent time in the evenings reading to Adolfo and Juan or playing games. At times, in the peaceful setting of his home, and with his nurturing presence, I felt like one of his children myself. He taught me about the real-estate market on the Spanish coast and asked me to move in with him. I loved Rafael.

At the end of the summer, when I was twenty-one, I wanted to stay in Spain and my mother supported the decision. She said it would only get ugly at home, with a divorce on the horizon and she didn't want me around to worry about her. Going back to school was pointless. I was learning the real-estate business and had someone to love me. Mostly, I was happy. "Every minute of happiness counts," my mother declared. I moved in with Rafael when my mother and Greg flew back to New York after Labor Day.

Rafael and I lived together for five years in a charming apartment in the old city of Marbella, called Orange Square. This section was protected from the creeping sterilization of development by strict zoning laws. There were narrow cobblestone streets where the terracotta roofs on one side almost touched those on the other; the cooking smells were wonderful and late at night I could hear guitar music from the tapas bar by the fountain. Early each morning Rafael got up, made breakfast for Adolfo and Juan, and laid out their clothes for school. After they left, we had breakfast together, then he went off to work. I went to the municipal market, a task I enjoyed—tasting the different cheeses, serrano hams, the various olives, and saying "hola!" to the fruit and vegetable vendors who knew me. Later, I'd meet Rafael at work.

An opportunity arose to purchase a piece of property in the cool of the mountains with wide views of the Mediterranean. I must have inherited my father's aggressive business sense and persuaded Rafael to purchase the land. We designed a complex of sixteen luxury houses and a swimming plaza. Rafael handled the legal negotiations and financing. My office was an on-site trailer from which I handled the construction team and sales. We worked until two o'clock in the afternoon, when all of Spain retires for siesta.

It was the antithesis of a New York City lifestyle. At six, we returned to work until nine P.M. Such was the business day in Spain. Once at home, Rafa, as I called him, cooked dinner and I did laundry. The four of us sat down to meals together. After dinner, it was homework time for the boys. Rafael supervised this and their bath time strictly.

I framed a collage of photographs we'd taken of ourselves in the mountains and hung it in the small foyer.

We dined out about once a week, or took a walk through the Puerto Banus. It was a simple life. Rafael was always an earnest parent. He didn't ask me to participate in the rearing of Adolfo and Juan. He didn't want me to take part in it, or to interfere. We spent time together, but he separated me from the care of the boys. Unquestionably, they came first. I felt neglected and "temporary." I was good to the children; I truly cared for them. I cooked once in a while and shopped, but there was always that separation and it grew larger every day. Adolfo and Juan were very polite and considerate of me. They picked up after themselves and helped me up the stairs with bundles, but there was no real affection. They were a family: Rafael, Adolfo, and Juan. I began to resent the boys.

Rafael wanted to marry me, but he didn't want any more children. I was twenty-six, and that was the first time I consciously thought of having a child. I could never have been a good stepmother to Juan and Adolfo. I had been an outsider and marriage wouldn't change that. I wanted a child of my own, and I missed my roots and my family. Though I loved Rafael, I finally went home to New York, not understanding that I was beginning to grow up and becoming ready, myself, to be a mother.

Today, considering my mother's singlemindedness in making Erica well and Greg's devotion to Stuart, I believe parenthood is what comes over you when you first hold your own child; knowing this life has been given to you to protect, you do so with ferocity. I think I had an inkling of this truth when I left Spain, but it was to take many years before I matured and had the ability to embrace it.

Chapter

6

*F*or each monthly menstrual cycle there is a 20 to 25 percent chance of pregnancy under ideal conditions. I was told this fact by my OB/ GYN. The percentages with in vitro fertilization are lower and are also dependent on the age and health of both prospective parents.

No one and no research can prepare you for what happens to a woman's emotional balance and her body when it is pumped up and manipulated by administered hormones. For me it was like being trapped in a volcano with a blazing fire beneath me. I pictured the upper edge of the crater but it was shrouded in fog. I knew my life would go on once I reached the top and climbed over the lip, but I was unable to see this far. I imagined myself time and again plunging into fiery depths and hauling myself upward because there was no-where else to go.

In 1986, when I left Rafael and came home from Spain, I was a stranger to the tough town of New York City. I was happy to see Jennifer. She greeted me with the exuberant warmth of our early childhood. We had exchanged only a few brief letters over the five years I was away. It wasn't because we didn't think of one another. It was, I believe, because for each of us it was a time of change, a time to free oneself of the past. And though our relationship had

had its ups and downs, the foundation my mother and Aunt Laurie had built for us remained firm.

Jennifer had left college after two years and was living alone in an apartment on Ninety-third Street and First Avenue. She had a lucrative job buying television time for advertisers, an expense account, and a closetful of business outfits. Over the years Jennifer had matured. She knew her mind and no longer looked to me to determine who she should be. (She was about to be married and asked me to be her maid of honor.)

She met Stephen Scheu through the media business. They greeted each other casually in the office, not because they'd been introduced but because physically they were drawn to each other. They just looked so good side by side. His six feet four inches complemented her height, and his black hair and full beard strikingly contrasted with her blond good looks. It was nice, for a change, to look up to a man, even standing by the water cooler. They began to meet each day for lunch. When the weather was warm, they'd have sandwiches in a rowboat and explore the lake at Central Park, throwing crusts of bread into the water and laughingly fighting over who had attracted the biggest fish.

Within six months of their meeting, Stephen was offered a sales manager position for a local TV station in Chicago, where he had grown up and where he was anxious to return. He had two little daughters living there with his ex-wife. He asked Jennifer to move with him. She was reluctant to pick up and go halfway across the country with someone she'd known less than a year.

More than anything, it was Jen's ties to Laurie that were keeping her in New York. Jennifer felt she and her mother had grown up together, they were locked into each other, and she was afraid the move would break their bonds. She thought of that afternoon in the hospital after Aunt Suzy had been so severely injured, how tightly I held her hand while she stroked my head. How lost I was without my mother and how in a flash fate can turn your life around.

"If you love me," she said to Stephen, "don't ask me to do this without marriage."

"Let's pack!" was his reply.

Laurie encouraged Jennifer to go. "You have to live your own life," she told her daughter. "Besides, with the air shuttle, it's only a short commute, not much longer than it takes to go downtown."

In October 1986, Jennifer and Stephen went to Chicago. She got a job, again selling media time. With gusto, Aunt Laurie embarked on plans for a January wedding. She decided on the landmark Puck Building in downtown New York City. It offered a vast space with no restrictions on the extravagant stage setting she, undoubtedly, would mastermind. Laurie and Jen collaborated on the telephone eight times a day and Jennifer flew to New York twice a month for visits and fittings of the spectacular bridal gown her mother was creating.

It was snowing lightly on January 9, Jennifer's wedding day. The two hundred guests stepped from winter's grayness into a lush, de-cadent Garden of Eden of fantasy-animal props and floral arrange-ments. The bridesmaids and I were dressed in glistening black. The bridal gown was a sheath of white satin, plunging low to Jennifer's more than ample bosom. Seed pearls and silken flower buds envel-oped the long train. Stephen looked dramatic in his tuxedo. Aunt Laurie gave the bride away. Her husband of four years, Stanley, beamed from the front row. Mother and daughter walked down the aisle side by side. Aunt Laurie wore a simple black velvet dress; her only accessory was her dazzling joy when she lifted Jennifer's veil and kissed her as Stephen came to usher his bride to the altar.

My mother gives a funny account of how Laurie met her husband. She was driving her famous gold Avanti through a tollbooth. An attractive man in a pristine powder-blue '57 T-Bird caught her eye from the next lane and smiled. She could see him following her in the rearview mirror, making signals to pull over. There was a diner at the next exit. He followed her off the exit and to the diner. She parked her car. He parked beside her.

"Do I know you?" she asked, flirt that she was.

"Please forgive me. I'm a car collector myself. I wanted to com-pliment you on the Avanti. I haven't seen one in good condition like yours. I'm Stanley," he said, standing tall and a bit awkward as he opened her car door.

They had coffee. He told her he owned a company that manufactured "soft" housewares.

She told him she was a designer.

Laurie took over the design department of Maycrest. She put her
hand to creating whimsical and geometric motifs for tablecloths,
place mats, and napkins. She went to Atlanta, Georgia, to the company's rug factory, and chose threads and drew patterns for the
braided rugs they manufactured. The company's gross income more
than doubled the first year. She "rearranged" Stanley to his greatest
advantage, having him grow a beard and mustache, which she manicured. She threw away his hair-stiffening gel and shopped with him
for a new wardrobe. She made Stanley a dapper man. He had become a rich man, too, with Laurie's help, and he was the first to
proclaim his wife's capabilities. Finally Laurie had found the life and
the respect she felt she had earned and she openly adored the man
who gave them to her.

I HAD BEEN in New York for six months and was living in a matchbox apartment on East Eighty-third Street that my friend Bonni had
vacated. If I were in Spain, I'd have been in one of my newly built
white houses watching fishing boats at sea. Instead, all I saw from
my window were fire escapes and bricks. The only thing growing
outside was a pile of blue recycling garbage bags. Bonni moved in
with her high-school sweetheart, Ken, figuring they would live in his
place after they were wed. Even Greg was engaged. He had skipped
college and was already a man, operating five restaurants in partnership with our father. Greg was twenty and his wife, Maxine, was
nineteen. Two kids, who loved and bickered together like puppies
since they were adolescents, knew their hearts with an enviable
clarity.

During the time I was in New York City, I obtained my real-
estate sales license, hoping it would lead me to work in development,
which I had enjoyed in Spain. Very quickly, I was disenchanted with
the files of women showing apartments up and down the length of

Manhattan. My social life was a string of tedious blind dates, which, for the most part, were more interviews than actual dates. I wanted a challenge. I liked doing business: it was in my blood and it suited me better than belonging to the throngs selling real estate. I made a down payment on a restaurant using profits Rafa and I shared from our business. After that payment and my living expenses, my bank account was practically nil.

I was in a hurry to open what would be a family-style Italian trattoria with a casual Mediterranean atmosphere. At last I had all my permits in order. I interviewed hundreds of prospective employees and trained a staff of fifty, which I needed for a restaurant that would accommodate 220 people. Now I set about the renovation. Jennifer offered to help me. How fortunate that she was in New York visiting Aunt Laurie at this time when I needed her. I plastered, Jennifer painted.

"How are you managing with Stephen's children?" I asked from atop a ladder.

"It's really no problem for me. I've been the baby long enough. Besides, if I let it upset me, it would threaten my relationship with Stephen."

"I didn't feel that way with Rafael's children. I wanted to, but I didn't."

"You weren't ready yet, Lollipop." Jen mixed a warm terra-cotta color, one that would flatter complexions by candlelight. The she sponged on the paint.

"You came together with Rafael because your family was splitting up. It was a safe haven. You loved him, but you looked to him to guide and protect you. He was all you had. You wanted *his* care, not to care for a family. That's just what you were escaping."

I continued to swirl the plaster. "My body has the instinct to open up, let someone in, to . . . nurture . . . such a corny word. My head beats it into submission. It's a real battle." Beads of dried plaster fell from my hair. "What a mess!" I spit the plaster flecks from my lips and wiped my eyes with my shirtsleeve. "It's not only about kids, Jen. Even with a man, I want to be the center of attention."

"Liza, I promise you, when you fall in love to marry, you will want to start your own family. Whatever or whoever belongs to your husband belongs to you. If it is children, you will love them but not enough to give up having children of your own. And, Liza, you will be at the center of attention because the family you create is the center."

"Jen, don't you resent the time his daughters take from you? I remember how you resented any distraction from your mother."

"That was different. I still feel the need for Mommy. Nothing, nothing has taken that from me. But I'm in a different place. With Stephen and the girls, I don't feel threatened. I just feel more love."

"I'm glad you and Stephen are happy."

"Yep. You have to give to get."

"*Your* mother tells you that, too?"

"Of course, they're sisters."

By three A.M., we had transformed the old catering hall into a Mediterranean dining fantasy. In the wee hours we opened a bottle of champagne and toasted my new restaurant and Jen's new marriage.

The restaurant filled the void I had felt since I returned to New York. I tirelessly worked eighteen hours a day, seven days a week, oftentimes crashing out on a few chairs put together, with a tablecloth as my blanket.

After three months I began to feel Sambuca had become a favorite in the neighborhood. People came in looking for me. "Where's Liza?" they asked if they didn't see me. I knew Elaine and Saul Cohen liked fresh mozzarella cheese and black olives in their house salad. Bob and Tom liked their martinis straight up with two olives when they arrived at their table. Mrs. Fisher liked to keep a plate over her pasta while she ate a little at a time. I knew who was well and who wasn't and would deliver meals across the street late at night and offer congratulations on graduations and births. I had created a small-town-neighborhood feeling in the middle of New York City because I took the time to know and care for my customers.

To my good fortune, an apartment on West Sixty-seventh Street facing Central Park West became available and I was able to afford the rent. I had a window from which I could appreciate the moonlit skyline late at night. Finally, I counted myself a success in New York City.

THE AROMAS OF COFFEE aroused me from my meditation.

"Liza, are you awake?" David asked, handing me my morning mug.

"I was dreaming."

"Lately, more times than not, you are far away."

"Contemplating the past gives me the strength I'll need for the future. I see that the women I respect most—my mother, Aunt Laurie, and Jennifer—have all had their own volcano to climb out of. They got a foothold and went forward. It gives me courage."

Chapter
7

*D*avid entered the in vitro commitment with optimism. I went with a loaded gun to my back. The ammunition was powerful: we wanted our biological child and the technology was there.

"Fifteen percent chance of having a baby," I said to David the night after the infertility doctor gave us the odds and we signed the consent form. "That would be a foolish bet."

"But if we win, it will be a treasure for a lifetime and all we will have lost is time . . . and sleep."

"And pain," I added. "I'm scared, David. I really am."

"I know, and if I could take the injections I would. I'll do anything to make it easier for you. I'm not asking you to do this, Liza. It is for both of us. It is your choice."

"I want our baby." There were tears in my eyes. "I'm sure of that, but I'm not sure I will survive the in vitro."

"You can stop whenever you want." He put his hand on my shoulder and turned me to face him. "Hear me, Liza, you can stop if you want."

I looked away. I trusted him. It was myself I doubted.

We arrived for our consultation at the infertility clinic at ten o'clock in the morning, half an hour early. Many of the patients in the waiting room appeared to be career women, hoping to start a family in their late thirties. I watched their blasé faces as they leafed through *Town & Country, Leisure,* and *Collectors' Art.* After the financial expense of in vitro, perhaps a few would still be able to afford the lifestyle showcased in those glossy magazines.

Why am I here? I asked myself. If not for David, I would have a baby the old fashioned way, flat on my back, being pleasured in the missionary position. We sat and waited in the claustrophobic green-painted room with cloisterlike windows and no hint of fresh air for over an hour. Finally we were called in to Dr. Blake's office. She was a middle-aged woman in a clinician's coat. She sat with a frozen smile behind her desk, with my history and David's chart from the urologist in front of her. My intuition told me she didn't look into our eyes as we spoke because she had seen, too often, in too many couples, this yearning for a child. She didn't want to risk getting personally involved and suffer their disappointment along with them. In a clinical voice, she explained step-by-step the procedure of in vitro fertilization. She told me to come back the next day when I would have a pap smear, electrocardiogram, a histogram, and general physical exam. David and I would each have HIV tests and full blood workups.

"Can't we start today?" I asked. "We've been anticipating this for so long. Let's just get on with it."

"All right." Her smile stretched. "First and most important, Liza, is to make certain your fallopian tubes are open. The tubes must be open in order to have an embryo transfer, which, you know, is part of the process. You understand, don't you?"

I nodded and David said yes.

"Very well." She pushed a button on her telephone. "Nancy, would you come in, please, we'll begin testing on Freilicher." The nurse came in.

"You can go with her, she'll draw blood for an AIDS test and then we'll do the histogram."

I looked at David; he squeezed my hand. I got up and followed the nurse. "What's a histogram?" I inquired of her.

"Don't worry, your husband will wait outside for you." She nodded, ignoring my question.

I undressed as I was told and went into the examining room. Nancy, the nurse, was eating from a bag of pretzel nuggets and picking her teeth with long red fingernails. I almost ran out of there, but another technician came in and took my blood and helped me onto the examination table, putting my feet in the stirrups. She did a vaginal sonogram and then the histogram: she inserted a catheter, which released fluid into my fallopian tubes. I watched the computer screen as the liquid traveled, indicating that the tubes were open. The pain was severe in my abdomen and I was crying. "Why didn't you tell me it would hurt?" I asked. I got no response.

The technicians moved about as if I weren't there, as if I were a pile of laundry. I was disappointed. I thought in vitro was the way out of this torment that had engulfed David and me. I thought we were special and our needs special. I knew it wasn't a surefire so-lution, but I went to the infertility clinic feeling hopeful. Now I had become a nonperson.

When it was over, I dressed quickly. David was waiting for me outside the door. "Follow me," the nurse said. "Here are your pre-scriptions." She handed me six little pieces of paper. "We'll go in here and I'll show you how to inject." All very cut-and-dried.

We entered a small cubicle with a tall cabinet containing many small drawers. She closed the green curtain.

"Take your underwear down to below your hips."

I hesitated.

"Open your trousers and lower your pants."

I did what she said. She took a red felt-tipped pen and marked a circle on my butt behind my hipbone.

"Alcohol and gauze pads are used to sterilize the area," she ex-plained, and swabbed the area.

She opened a drawer in the beige cabinet and took out three different-size needles. One was long and as fat as a knitting needle. She demonstrated how to fill the syringes and make a fountain of liquid by pushing the stopper to get out any air bubbles. I thought she was going to inject it into that bull's-eye she'd drawn, and started to cry anew.

David took my hand. I looked so ridiculous, crying, with a big red circle drawn on my naked butt.

"I'm not going to stick you," she said matter-of-factly, without any sympathy for my fear. "You'll have boxes of disposable syringes," she told us. "Unwrap the individual syringe and attach one of the disposable needles. Each medication requires a different-size needle, so be sure you note the size written on the wrapper. After you prepare the dosage, switch to a fresh needle so it is really sharp. See here where I put the red circle? Put your hands on your hipbones and your thumb to the back of your hip. The meaty area there, about an inch in circumference, is the correct injection site. Change hips each night. Put alcohol on your skin and dry it with a sterile gauze pad. Remember—before you start, have the injection ready. David, you will pinch that fleshy area with one hand to tighten the skin. With your other hand you will inject with a quick flick of your wrist, using strength. The skin is tough. Push the plunger to release the medication and withdraw the syringe. Use a clean gauze pad with alcohol to swab the area clean, using pressure. Then cover it for a few hours with a Band-Aid. Practice on an orange."

She handed each of us a piece of fruit from a small refrigerator. "David, you'll have to practice the most, you'll be administering the medication." She demonstrated how he was to flick his wrist to get the momentum needed to push the needle through the skin. "Think of it as a dart. You'll be using different-size needles. Some are quite thick. I'll give you a video to watch before you do it."

I looked at that needle. "Forget it. There's no way I'm doing this."

David took my hand again. "Liza, it'll be okay. Come on."

We were given a schedule, alcohol pads, and a start-up amount of syringes and medicine.

"Isn't this exciting?" she said in a high, squeaky voice, as she handed me the package and a video. "This video should help you. Aren't you excited?" she repeated, perhaps in a vain attempt to be uplifting.

"No." I was crying. "It's terrifying."

I don't remember if David went to work after we left the hospital. He took me home and I went to sleep.

We were due to start the injections the following Monday, pending all the blood-test results. I wanted to approach IVF on my own terms and spent hours in Barnes & Noble's browsing the women's-health section. I bought eight books on in vitro and infertility, wanting to know as much as I could. I thought such information would make me feel comfortable, but what I was really looking for was another person's personal story. I was looking for something positive I could latch on to. In all the books I read, I found only one that offered anyone's personal experience. It was a mere two paragraphs long. The in vitro process was, as I feared, a lonely, cold experience.

Chapter

8

*T*he day of the first injection I called David at the office to make sure he'd be home well before eight. This was the designated hour because the shots had to be twelve hours apart, morning and evening. Of course, I didn't need to remind him. We didn't think of anything else.

Our lovely bedroom was transformed into a laboratory. My antique brass bed and lace curtains, my Wedgwood-blue-painted walls clashed with the tray that held the equipment for the injection. I had put the tray on my vanity table and hidden my collection of perfume bottles beneath the white lace skirt of the table. When David came home we watched the instructive video for the tenth time.

"David, can you really do this? Are you sure you can do it? Aren't you scared?"

I was to get one shot of Lupron, which suppressed the pituitary gland, in one arm, and in the other heparin, the blood thinner, prescribed by my hemotologist as a prophylactic for my particular condition.

"Are you ready?" David asked. He had filled a syringe and now had it poised in the air.

"No. No. No. Wait. Okay . . . go . . . no—wait! Aren't we sup-

posed to ice it first? Yes. Someone said ice. Wait." I ran to the
kitchen and bought fifteen minutes icing my arms.

"Okay," I said with conviction, back in the bedroom, closing my
eyes and scrunching up my face as I sat on the bed, gripping the
head board. David kissed the top of my head and calmly injected
the Lupron into my arm.

It hurt, probably more than it would have if I hadn't been so
tense. We lacked experience, so the whole process of injecting was
slow. Faster was better. Later, we found out that icing makes the
skin get hard and constricted, so it is more difficult to pierce with
the needle. It is amazing that I wasn't told these simple things at the
clinic. Eventually, I'd take a hot shower to open the pores and soften
my skin. I'd want to stay in the shower, where it was warm and
safe and private. David always knocked on the door. "It's almost
eight o'clock, come on, let's get it over with so we can have dinner
and relax."

I'd be so hot from the shower and sweaty from nerves that after
it was over, I had to shower again.

Within a few days, I began to feel the effects of the Lupron. The
nurse was right when she said it would give me a feeling of doom.
David and I would be alone having dinner at home or in a restaurant
and for no reason I would start to cry. If the light shifted, a shadow
passed, or I heard the honk of flying geese at our beach house, where
I sought escape and happiness, I was filled with despair. The sight
of my once blooming garden, lying dormant for the winter, sent me
into fits of weeping. And women running after children, or pushing
baby carriages in the park, a ball being tossed, plunged me into dark
pits of depression.

I didn't know myself. I was useless at work, and behaved out of
character, snapping at customers who knew my problem and wished
me well. These longtime customers, whom I considered friends, in-
furiated me with their kindness. To shake hands with Mr. Coniff
because his wife had a baby was difficult; when he wished me luck
it gave me pain. I couldn't continue. How would I tell David?

I called David's urologist, as a source of help, maybe because I had
had more conversations with him than with any other doctor and he

seemed most sympathetic to David and me, as individuals. I was crying. "I can't go through with this. No one knows if this will work and I'm putting poison into my body. Maybe it's not meant to be."

I thought he might suggest an alternative to IVF. "Why can't David's sperm that you retrieve be inseminated vaginally to fertilize the egg that I normally produce each month as would be done with donor sperm?" I asked him.

"Because, Liza, David's sperm is immature and couldn't penetrate the egg. With David's sperm, your eggs must be harvested and fertilized in the laboratory by a technician. You know all this, Liza."

He suggested I once again speak to the infertility psychologist, Patricia Greene.

As always, she was direct, honest, and well informed. Patricia explained the process of in vitro fertilization to us in human terms, being very specific about the side effects of the medications. The one thing she said that remained in my mind and helped me was to think of IVF as a means to an end. She told me the doom and despair meant the Lupron was working, that it was not a permanent "condition."

"Liza, you must understand that Lupron puts your body into a medically induced menopause. Your hormone levels have been greatly lowered. That's one cause of the hot flashes and sweats you experience. Don't be alarmed if you haven't been sexually aroused. That, too, is a reaction to Lupron."

It was true, David and I had not had sex—even before I began the cycle. From the time we started trying to get pregnant, I considered sex an offensive medical procedure. I had seen the surgical dressings and stitches after David's reconstructive surgery and regarded both our bodies as infertility laboratories. There was no chance of eroticism. David, I know, felt the same way; however, we didn't talk about it, for which I was glad. He never touched me as he did before we were aware of our infertility problem.

With our guards up against acknowledging our feelings of inadequacy, there was no chance of surmounting the sexual barrier. We had forgotten that sex is not solely a means for reproduction, it is an expression of love. Had we been secure and able to regard sex as revitalizing, we would have found comfort in each other's arms. But self-confidence is the first victim of Lupron's attack. I was becoming dysfunctional—quick to cry, nervous, rude, short-tempered.

Patricia told me, "Liza, your emotional sensitivity is related to Lupron. When you stop the medicine, you will be the same women you were before."

"No. It's me. They make me feel as if I don't count as a person. The doctors and nurses treat me so coldly, without any dignity or compassion or humanity."

"Liza, many patients have the same complaints. Try calling other women you know who are going through it or have done IVF. It really makes people feel better to express their feelings to others who share the experience."

I wanted to believe all that Patricia explained, that these feelings of anger and rejection and disgust at the lack of civility in the world were not emanating from me but were induced by the Lupron, but I didn't believe it. Nothing seemed real to me. I didn't know this person I had become. Both David and I were emotional strangers, to each other and to ourselves.

I felt most alone when I was in the waiting room of the IVF clinic with the other women. The unperturbed faces of these well-heeled New Yorkers seemed to tell me that getting pregnant was a business problem to be overcome. There was no common ground between me and them; in my mind, they were not experiencing the same torment. I felt I was being victimized.

Eventually, out of self-preservation, I heeded Patricia's advice and started speaking to my neighbor and two other women who were doing an IVF cycle. Patricia was right: it did feel good to talk to other people, though at first it was painful and difficult to expose what I had kept private for so long. I discovered they too felt IVF was a cold lonely process and had their own angst. We began to care about each other's progress. It became important to check in each day and speak to others about their reactions to the medication, or how they were dealing with their lives in the world apart from in vitro. They were sympathetic, and so was I. These relationships took away the feeling of being alone and were my greatest support.

MY MOTHER HAD BECOME a stone sculptor. She worked almost daily at the Sculpture Centre Studio on East Sixty-ninth Street and Aunt Laurie took two mornings off from work to meet her there. Laurie made abstract forms that coiled like intestines. My mother did large torsos, which seemed to strive to achieve her own limited activity and appeared to be caught in motion. On that morning of January 9, 1989, one year after Jennifer's wedding, Laurie was complaining.

"Suzy, I don't know if I can work today. I've had a pain in my back and chest. I haven't been able to sleep in a week."

"It's no wonder; you've been carting around those heavy rocks for the garden. Why don't you get help? Spring is a long way away. You must have pulled a muscle or wrenched your back. Go to the doctor anyway."

On January 9, 1989, Jennifer was in her office happily accepting congratulations on her one-year wedding anniversary. That evening she and Stephen planned to celebrate at an elegant restaurant in Chicago. When the phone rang in her office, she wasn't surprised to hear her mother's voice, but it sounded tight, strained. Something was wrong. Jennifer insisted she tell.

"I went to the doctor for that pain. I . . . I have cancer . . ."

Jennifer couldn't catch her breath. Laurie's husband, Stanley, got on the telephone; he sounded as if he had been shot in the stomach. Jennifer was sobbing and screaming. She couldn't speak. Stephen came to pick her up. He brought her suitcase and put her on a plane for New York.

Stanley called Jack. When he arrived at the apartment, he was bewildered. He had never seen his mother sick and it made him angry.

Jennifer stayed in the city for two weeks until a diagnosis was reached and she learned of the possible treatments. The prognosis was favorable. It was lymphoma and was treatable. Laurie prepared herself to do battle.

She continued to work. We had luncheons together whenever possible—my mother and I, Laurie and Jennifer. Stanley and Laurie came to my restaurant at night with Jen and my mother would meet them. We rallied together. As a family we were going to prevail. We refused to allow our collective life to be devastated; we continued all our activities together and didn't become morose over the present, but spoke of the future. And we laughed. Aunt Laurie and my mother, the sisters, with their own way of looking at life, kept our spirits seemingly high. In battle, it is their doctrine: if you go in with a strong constitution, you have the upper hand.

Privately, my mother drank a glass of wine each night to help her get through it, and when I saw her in the morning her eyes were red and swollen. She wouldn't talk about her appearance and she wouldn't say the name of the disease that was our adversary. She just wanted to be there and do for her sister whatever she could, and so did I.

EVERY DAY FOR A WEEK, then every other day for two weeks, I had to go to the hospital for blood tests and sonograms. Still, I could not sit there quietly like the other women, appearing unruffled, looking at *The New York Times* and magazines. I was angry and frustrated and impatient. I resented having to be there. I would pace around, change my seat, make phone calls, and watch the waiting list. I hoped to hear my name called and dreaded it at the same time. Every day a different person called me.

"Lisa Frolisher . . ."

Couldn't they even get my name right?

"Freilicher—Liza Freilicher," I said through clenched teeth.

I went into the changing room, donned the paper gown I was given, and then I would "sit there" as instructed. Freezing, I sat for twenty minutes. Another stranger came in and called me by another mispronunciation of my name. They did the sonogram without so much as looking me in the face. "Okay, go into the lab down the hallway to your right, for your blood test. Someone will call you tonight with your dosages." I knew the procedure: every day the medication dosage must be determined based on the hormone levels in the blood and the measured growth of the egg-producing follicles that had been examined by a vaginal sonogram. Simply, dosage is determined by the combined factors of follicle size and levels of hormones in the blood.

After the early hospital visit, I was not free to pursue my life. I was on the telephone, endlessly tracking down drugstores that carried the medications I needed. Pergonal, it turned out, was difficult to find. An alternative to Metrodin, Pergonal is the hormone that hyperstimulates the ovaries to produce more eggs than they would produce during a normal cycle. One pharmacist said Pergonal was so hard to come by because it was made from the urine of nuns—virgins who had not yet built up antibodies to spermatozoa. I didn't know if there was truth in this, but there was certainly humor, and for me, humor was rare. I had a long list of pharmacists who could possibly carry this hormone. One had six ampules, one had eight; one was expecting more the next day. I began to hoard Pergonal. Often a druggist forgot to include the syringes. He'd have to call the infertility clinic for the correct prescription. I often waited an hour or so in pharmacies around Manhattan for the prescription to be called in. I cried, from frustration, in more drugstores than I can remember. At length, I'd call my friends; perhaps they had leftover ampules or syringes. I became superstitious. If one woman became pregnant, I was anxious to get my hands on her stash.

Besides the hospital, I was sent to labs to do special blood tests due to my previous blood-clotting problem, which was, hopefully, under control. In vitro is a full-time job; in fact, many women are told by their physicians at the outset, "Either you have a job or you try to have the baby—you can't do both."

Not everyone can put his or her job on hold. For me, this was the first time in nine years that I just couldn't get to the restaurant. My whole day was spent dealing with IVF-related responsibilities; the evening ended with my round of telephone calls.

"How does your husband give you the shot?"

"Do you hate your husband because he gives you the shot?"

One of the women told me about "Resolve" meetings. These are gatherings held in various clinics where guest speakers, usually infertility doctors, endocrinologists, or embryologists reach out for an hour or so and answer questions. Usually, they are questions that other doctors had tried to answer before, but couldn't answer because there was not enough data to support a definite answer. The meetings were informative, not support groups like Alcoholics Anonymous. They told of upcoming experiments and theories, new drugs and programs. The technology in the field of infertility was changing so rapidly that in six months many things relevant today could be obsolete.

Within a week after my first injections, I was feeling very uncomfortable. I was emotionally and physically hyperstimulated. My stomach was distended; after the third week I looked four months pregnant and couldn't stand up straight. I was able to wear only two skirts, both of which had soft elastic waistbands, and I alternated between them. My skin hurt. I continued on the drugs and became more and more distended and uncomfortable. Secretly I marveled at my aunt Laurie's stamina and tried to fathom what had made her go on.

Laurie started oral chemotherapy in the spring of 1989 and bought a big hat. She felt well and looked healthy. The tumor in her neck had gotten smaller. My mother and I spent a lot of time with her while she rested in the apartment, and we kept the conversation away from illness. I became the featured topic.

"So, Lollipop, when are you and Ben getting married?" Ben was a fine Israeli dentist I had been dating for two years. Laurie respected and liked him and thought we could get through the obstacles of being from two different cultures. "He can support you. If you have love and he makes you happy, what else do you need?"

I couldn't answer. I knew my aunt's illness was life threatening. I wanted with all my heart to make her happy. I knew that my being on my way to marriage and starting a family would give her peace.

Aunt Laurie was on her bed, resting against the pillows in her dimly lit bedroom. My mother sat in a chair by her side and I was lying across the bottom of the bed among a mess of fashion magazines.

"Liza, what do you need to make up your mind about Ben?"

"I need what Jen has with Stephen and what you and Stanley have. The conviction of being a couple, of being one. Ben and I have such different ideas about what family means—what a woman's role is in the family. I don't want to be a baby machine. I think that's all he expects of his wife. I don't want to give up Sambuca."

"Haven't you two discussed this?"

"Yes, but his answer is vague. He says he wants children. When he asks if I do, I say yes. And then he tells me in conclusion that we have no problem. I'm not convinced."

"You can't be happy this way. One minute yes and one minute no. Don't you think it would be best to decide and give that decision a chance? Get engaged, and see how that works. You don't have to get married right away."

What she said made sense; I had been procrastinating. "You mean I should either see how I feel with him or without him, and spend more time exploring our differences."

Laurie reached out and touched her sister's hand. "What do you think, Suzy?"

"Whatever you decide, Liza, I'll agree to. It's how you feel. But this way, you haven't given yourself a chance either way."

Aunt Laurie closed her eyes. "I want you to be happy, and settled. I love you as my own, La. Happiness and health is all that matters in life. Settle it. Don't waste a moment of happiness."

She paused, then turned to my mother. "Suzy, do you remember how we used to daydream about our children being raised together?"

My mother smiled. "We had no aunts or uncles or cousins. We wanted to give you and Jennifer a big family to surround yourselves with."

Aunt Laurie took her sister's hand in hers. "And very soon we will see another generation."

With the urging of Aunt Laurie and the promise from my mother that she would support my decision either way, I felt confident. "I'll tell Ben, yes. I feel better already. What a relief to finally decide, and know where I'm going."

I loved my aunt. It hurt me to see her suffer. I knew her strength and wanted to give her hope. Aunt Laurie saw Jennifer was happy and would soon have children and she saw that I was settled. It gave her a sense of harmony to see life going on and to be a part of it. It was up to me to maintain that harmony.

*A*fter four weeks, I was ready to be prepared for my egg retrieval.
The doctor who examined me told me I would get an HCG (human
chorionic gonadotropin) shot that night to release the eggs from the
follicles. I was to take the HCG shot and come to the hospital thirty-
four hours later, allowing time to be prepped. The retrieval must
occur thirty-six hours after the shot, because HCG releases the follicles from the ovaries in thirty-six hours. Any other time would not
be ideal for the viability of the eggs.

It was a big needle and the medicine burned as it went in. Plus,
my butt was sore from weeks of injections. Every day David alternated the injection site; nevertheless, by now we were working over
old bruises.

We arrived at Mount Sinai ambulatory unit at six o'clock in the
morning. A nurse told us to wait in the main waiting room. Dirty,
bloody tissues littered the floor; people were sick and coughing. I
had to fill out many forms and wait . . . wait . . . wait to speak to
the doctor. The receptionist told me, "The doctor won't come out,
you must wait until the procedure to speak to your doctor." Eventually, I was weighed, given an eye test, and had my temperature
taken—all hospital policy. After more repetitive questions, I was
told to have a seat . . . wait.

"Leeza Freilger."

I was escorted to a locker room and given paper pajamas, cap and shoes, and returned to the waiting room, feeling dehumanized in that paper wrapping. David and I sat together holding hands, saying nothing. A man dressed in hospital scrubs the same color as my paper rolled up a gurney and said, "Get up on here."

"Can't I walk down?"

"No. It's hospital policy."

"I'd like to see the doctor. I want to talk to her before I go into surgery."

"Don't worry, you'll see the doctor in the OR."

"Can my husband come with me?"

"No, it's hospital policy."

"Wait. I want to go to the bathroom." But the urge left once I got there. I climbed onto the gurney, holding the tears back. David kissed me. I was wheeled through double swinging doors and more double doors, all the while becoming more frightened and feeling like a piece of meat on a wagon. The attendant stopped and parked me by the wall in a hallway, adding to a long line of occupied gurneys. I stared at the ceiling until the glaring lights made my eyes burn at which point I closed them. Something jolted the gurney. My eyes popped open. I was being pushed into the OR. No one spoke to me. They removed my paper gown, put me on the operating table, and covered me with a sheet.

"Where's the doctor?" No response.

They strapped my hands at my sides and my feet in the stirrups. Six people were poking my arms, looking for my veins to begin an IV. I couldn't escape. I panicked. I was drowning in a sea of white-coated technicians.

The anesthesiologist came in and asked me the same questions I'd answered before. I was shaking with cold and sweating. My eyes must have been wild.

"We'll find you a blanket."

I was looking around the room—the big round lights, the IV pole, monitoring screens, people carrying trays and wheeling tables in and out in silence. The scene had an eerie, surrealistic aura. It was strange to think David and I were trying to have a child—the most basic and primitive of acts. I was terrified to be put to sleep and just leave my body there on the table, with no control over what was done to me. Awake, I could watch out for myself. Did they know why I was there? Would they mix me up with someone else?

The doctor arrived at the last minute. "Relax. It will be over in a few minutes. Relax."

"Why do I have to be put to sleep if the eggs are retrieved vaginally? I'd rather be awake. I don't want anesthesia." I struggled against the straps holding my arms to the table.

"Relax now, Liza. You have to be asleep. I have to locate and withdraw delicate egg follicles from your ovaries. You can't be awake; the procedure is precise and we can't damage the eggs."

The anesthesiologist was feeling my arm. I felt the needle stick. Someone covered me with the long-awaited blanket. I was quivering.

"Relax your legs."

AUNT LAURIE WAS NOT feeling better. She was not responding to the chemotherapy as expected. The doctor told her, as well as Jennifer and Stanley on their last visit, that the tumor had grown and the cancer had spread to her intestines.

Jennifer spent most of her weeks in New York with her mother. She would fly to Chicago for an occasional weekend to be with her husband, but it was a great emotional effort for her to do so and she resented the obligation.

Jennifer and Stanley took Aunt Laurie to various oncologists for opinions and learned about controversial treatments being given around the world. They were tireless in their search for a cure. Laurie's New York specialist started her on a course of more aggressive chemotherapy.

In May 1989, Stanley took Laurie to Chicago, seeking an alternative to standard chemotherapy. She had lost weight. When she looked in the mirror, she no longer slapped her hips. "Be careful what you wish for, you never know how you may get it," she said, trying to hold on to her sense of humor.

Jennifer prepared the guest room of her and Stephen's house and Stanley and Laurie moved in while Laurie went to a research clinic in Chicago. It was to be the first of many experimental treatments, which would eventually take Stanley, Jennifer, and Laurie to places like Canada and Boston. In late December, Mother and I met them in Houston.

Jennifer couldn't deny how sick her mother was. She didn't plan to have kids for three more years, until she was thirty. But she wouldn't refuse her mother a grandchild. All she thought of was "I have to get pregnant."

She told me how her mother stood outside the bedroom door and called "Go, baby, go" while Jennifer and Stephen were making love, and how afterward, with Stephen still in the bed, Laurie would come in to rub her belly, saying, "Give me a baby girl."

Pregnancy became Jennifer's single focus.

Stephen said nothing. At this time he felt like he was not a high priority in his wife's life. He wanted a baby with Jennifer, and knew how important it was to her at this time. It was strange to have his mother-in-law around as a cheerleader, but since the start of this tragic illness, nothing was usual.

Jennifer knew she had conceived. She said she willed it to happen. Two weeks later she was awake at 5:30 A.M. to take the pregnancy test. It was positive. She woke her mother to tell her. "It's a good omen. All is going to be okay."

Jennifer and her mother talked and talked about the baby. They discussed every detail. Laurie called her grandchild by the name Jennifer had chosen. "Dakota. Oh, my baby girl, I know just how you will look—blue eyes, white skin, brown hair. And she'll call me Namsy. I'll take her to fabulous places and we'll do wonderful things together. Just like Auntie Mame. You will have a daughter, Jennifer, and you will love her as I love you and she will always give you joy."

Greg and Maxine had their first baby in August. When I saw my brother holding his son in the nursery, it created a connection for me I never experienced before. His heart was in his eyes when he looked at his child, and since then I always look at Stuart with the love I remember seeing in his father's eyes. Aunt Laurie was very weak but found the strength to drive with my mother to Greg's house in Long Island so she could hold her baby nephew.

Jennifer was five months pregnant in October 1989. She left her job and moved to New York to be with her mother.

In December, Jennifer and Stanley took Aunt Laurie to a private institute in Houston. Mother and I flew to Texas to be with her. The radical treatment she was receiving there was showing signs of success. It allowed Aunt Laurie to be well enough to be in Chicago with Jen when the baby, a C-section, was born as scheduled. Aunt Laurie was there in the delivery room holding Jen's hand when Stephen placed her granddaughter in her arms. Dakota is blue-eyed, with white skin and soft brown hair, just as Aunt Laurie had pictured her. It was good to share.

Laurie's battle with cancer was exhausting and ravaged her body, yet she was empowered by joy to see her healthy grandchild.

After four days, Stanley took his wife back to New York. It was partly at her insistence; she wanted Jennifer's life with her husband and their new baby to be as normal as possible.

Being alone now, for the first time since that phone call of January 9, 1989, a year ago, Jennifer thought about herself. She thought about being a mother and what it meant. She almost felt guilty knowing she had to divide her attention between her child and her mother. There wasn't enough time for both. But her daughter, peacefully sucking at her breast, told her where her allegiance would lie for the rest of her life. It was, Jennifer reflected, nature's way of taking care of itself, that protective instinct that overwhelms a female when her milk flows. She was dozing, glad to be alone and connected to "Kodie."

"You have a loving family." The words were spoken by the girl in the next bed. Jennifer had barely been aware of her over the past four days. The girl had had no visitors and slept most of the time when she wasn't nursing her baby son. "You don't remember me.

I've seen you at the gym. I'm Hilary Steele. Your mother is brave. She's very ill, isn't she?"

Jennifer nodded.

"My mother, too."

"That's why you're alone?"

"I'm not alone anymore." She marveled at her baby's clenched fists. "I have him. I've named him Michael."

Jennifer and Hilary, in that brief period of intimacy, exchanged their stories. It was amazing that two people of the same age with such different backgrounds could end up at the same place in life at the same time.

Hilary came from an extremely affluent family. Her mother was a socialite and not available in the role of mother. "Daughter" was a title with no more connection to either of her parents than the fleeting glimpse of figures coming and going behind closed doors. Hilary was cared for by a nanny to whom she transferred all her love. It was a childhood without any security or structure, and though she felt loved by her nanny she saw herself isolated and apart from other children, who spoke possessively of their parents. Hilary married quickly with dreams of creating a perfect family of her own. It healed the wound temporarily by yielding a son. But even as she lay in the hospital with Michael at her breast, she knew the marriage would not last.

And Jennifer, who had nothing but love and who was her mother's "Princess" was here, equally alone in the world.

She and Hilary left the hospital with a deep bond and mutual empathy. They spent their days going to the park or the gym or just having coffee in each other's kitchen with their children. They shared a private dimension. It was their strength. Hilary never succumbed to despair; she picked herself up and barreled forward. She faced single parenthood as an opportunity to transcend the neglect of her childhood and didn't feel victimized. Jennifer leaned on Hilary's strength, and Hilary, in turn, leaned on Jennifer for stability and a sense of family.

I WAS CONFUSED when I awoke in the recovery room. My mouth was dry. My stomach kept cramping and I was dizzy. I asked a nurse if she could please bring me some water.

"First go to the bathroom."

"Where's David? How is my husband?"

"You'll see him shortly. He's fine."

While my eggs were being retrieved, David was in the adjacent operating room having a testicular biopsy to extract his sperm. He had been calm about undergoing the procedure, but nervous about the outcome, wondering whether his sperm would be mature enough to fertilize my eggs.

The nurse sat me up slowly and helped me into the bathroom, pushing the IV pole that was still attached to my arm. I was afraid it would be painful to urinate but it wasn't.

I came back and sat down in a wheelchair. "Please, can I speak to the doctor. I want to know how many eggs were retrieved." No response.

I was wheeled into another recovery room, where I saw David. He was groggy and still lying on a gurney.

He smiled. "They retrieved twelve eggs and the urologist believes he got good sperm. The embryologist is doing ICSI in the lab. Tomorrow we'll know how many became embryos with good cell division."

We had arrived at the hospital at six A.M., and left at five P.M. David's surgery was one hour and so was mine, yet with the preop test, releases to be filled out, the surgery, and recovery, we had spent eleven hours, the entire day, there.

David and I helped each other into a cab. Both Greg and my mother had offered to pick us up, but we felt it would be easier just to get a cab; the fewer people, the less confusion. I could barely walk and David moved very slowly. He was in pain, I knew, but he didn't complain. We went home and got into bed and slept, anxious for tomorrow when we'd hear how the fertilization was progressing.

Chapter

10

*I*n the morning, I called the clinic. I tried the doctor and I tried to speak to the embryologist.

"The doctor's not available. Call back," was the cold response to each inquiry.

I did—the results weren't in. "Call back."

I called back. "Fertilization appears good. Tomorrow we will know more."

David and I spent three days doing nothing but speculating futilely. Our life was being decided by the embryologist monitoring the cell division of the embryos.

A question arose about whether the doctors should do assisted hatching. The embryologist explained that assisted hatching involves cracking the egg before transferring the embryo, to make it easier for the egg to adhere to the uterine wall. The egg must adhere to the uterine wall for a successful implantation that could lead to pregnancy. No one knew for sure if assisted hatching was advantageous. It was experimental. It seemed to me in vitro was experimental as well. The infertility doctor and the embryologist decided to do the assisted hatching on all of the six embryos that would be transferred.

Decisions continued to crop up. Should I continue on the blood thinner, heparin? My doctor said to stay on it because I still had the hormones in my system that caused a potential risk of clotting. Other hematologists recommended going off heparin because, should extensive bleeding occur, my blood would not clot and hemorrhage could result. It was decided that I should continue on the heparin.

After three days, the embryos would be transferred into my uterus. I was still very bloated and very uncomfortable. I was taking antibodies to prevent any infection during the procedure and had started progesterone injections to thicken and make my uterine wall more apt for the embryos to adhere to. It was a thick, difficult shot. I dreaded going back to the ambulatory unit, a place for truly sick people and accident victims. I didn't belong there. I tried to think positively: tomorrow I would have an embryo growing in my body that would be my baby. My baby. My baby. I tried to think positively, but I didn't believe it. My baby. I tried to focus on the positive . . . my baby.

Again, I was back in the operating room, where I was asked my name and to identify the name on the test tubes of embryos. I was prepped and put in position on the table. The embryos were loaded into a catheter. I watched those embryos—my babies—being nestled into my uterus on the sonogram screen. I was squeezing the hands of the nurses on either side of me. I wanted to be hopeful and to feel pregnant with those embryos inside me.

It was incredible to watch, to actually be able to see, what I prayed would be the beginning of life inside of me, and then to realize that man, with all his medicine and technology, could only do so much. I knew all I could do was hope and pray one of those embryos would be my baby, healthy and strong in my arms, in my life. It was frightening to be filled with so much hope without a promise and it was also exhilarating.

It was a short procedure. I was told to remain lying down for half an hour.

David came in, smiling. Was I, would I be pregnant? These were the questions I read in his face.

"Okay, Liza, you can go now," the nurse said, putting out her hand to help me up.

I was surprised that they just let me walk away. I didn't give her my hand. I wanted to stay longer to be on the safe side. I was afraid to move. I stayed until an orderly came into the room and began to mop the floor in preparation for another patient.

I stayed in bed for two days while David was at work. I was afraid to get up even to go to the bathroom. Greg came and brought or cooked dinner for us each night, and during the day my mother lay next to me on the bed while we watched videos. Jennifer called to give me encouragement.

"Think positively, La La. Lie back with your legs in the air as I did. Picture those embryos and will them to hug your womb. Talk to them."

"Jen, you make me feel good. To talk to them gives them life. I'm glad you had Dakota first. I know how hard you tried for her, how you set your mind to it. It wasn't easy for you." I had no resentment of Jennifer for having her baby so easily. God knows she was suffering a greater heartache. Neither did I resent Maxine and Greg the ease of Stuart's birth. I resented no one. I just wanted this quest that David and I had embarked upon to be successful.

For two weeks, I just waited, not believing, not thinking, still taking my injections and waiting. I tried, at night, before I went to sleep, to visualize being pregnant. I was numb and felt emotionally battered. My body hurt. I was still bloated, tender, and uncomfortable. The day before the pregnancy test, I saw some staining. I called the doctor.

"Give it another day," she said. "It doesn't necessarily mean anything."

Since the transfer, I knew there was always the possibility of my period coming. Each time I went to the bathroom I was scared to look. I choked down my sneezes so as not to jolt my insides. The doctor said, "Don't worry," but that's what my life was about. The thought of the cycle not working was devastating. When I saw the blood, I had an overwhelming desire to escape my body, which had failed me.

"Don't worry, it doesn't mean anything," the doctor said.

I wanted to rip her throat out. "What do you mean it doesn't mean anything? Then why is it happening?"

During those weeks since the transfer, I continued the progesterone and heparin shots as I was told. I saw the blood, knew what it meant, and still I had to pump what I considered poison into my body. I knew I wasn't pregnant. What had been difficult before was even more disgusting now.

Very early the next day I went for the long awaited blood test to determine pregnancy. I gave the laboratory my mother's telephone number and went to her apartment to wait for the results.

I lay on the sofa with my head on my mother's lap. She stroked my hair the way that always comforted me, but I couldn't close my eyes. The telephone was all I could think about. It sat on the white table amid framed photos of me, Erica, and Greg, and one of Aunt Laurie and Mother in wide straw hats.

"I remember," I said, "how simple life was in Spain. Rafa took care of me, I had no worries. I didn't need to concern myself with having children, and if I wanted to feel maternal, I could have cultivated that feeling and bestowed it on his boys."

"But that isn't what your wanting a child is about. That was the reason you left Rafael, wasn't it?"

"Yes," I said tentatively, "and I missed you."

"But, La, you love David, the two of you want this child to be your legacy, as my children are mine and Laurie's children are hers. I know you're frightened now; don't let your doubts take over your mind. Stay focused. You'll accomplish this. You've been thoroughly examined, you are fine, and produce healthy eggs. We'll have a child and it will be your own."

"Mom, I'm not pregnant now," I said, my eyes riveted to the telephone. "I'm staining more heavily."

She stroked my hair.

We waited and I thought of the past, which is ever present with me, during Laurie's illness when all reasonable hope was gone, and still my mother, my aunt Laurie, Jennifer, and I held on.

PASSOVER CAME LATE in March of 1990. Laurie wasn't able to go out anymore. Stanley and Jennifer stayed with her and administered her medications. The doctors could no longer help.

Aunt Laurie asked her sister if she could "please" have the seder at her apartment. Those two, no matter what, they kept to their traditions: Laurie had Thanksgiving, Suzy had Passover.

Mom made the turkey and pot roast. Erica was up and out early, an uncommon event, and stood on line at the bakery for chocolate-dipped macaroons. I arranged the traditional seder plate with the lamb-shank bone, horseradish, burned egg, and parsley—all the symbols of Passover. Maxine brought the chicken soup and matzo balls, praying they wouldn't be "like rocks" this year. Ben, my dentist boyfriend, picked up everything in his car and delivered it to Laurie's apartment.

Nothing was left undone when we arrived. Miriam, my mother's aide, eagerly went into the kitchen to organize the meal. The table by the window was open wide and set with Aunt Laurie's elegant crystal stemware, and Limoges china.

Aunt Laurie sat at the head of the table flanked by her children. She was unmistakably radiant. Her gray silk belly skirt, camisole, and cardigan were enhanced by a delicate coral-and-diamond necklace. In one ear she wore an earring, an heirloom that had been her grandfather's stickpin, and in the other a diamond stud. Erica was seated next to Jack. She was petite, with a perfect, curvaceous body. Her thick honey-colored hair matched Jack's. Somewhere in our family there was a good-hair gene. Next to Jack was Greg and Max and Stuart, in his baby seat. Stephen sat beside Jennifer with Dakota in her arms. Stanley was at the far end of the table facing Laurie, Ben, Mom, and me. Grandma Reese was there, not fully understanding the gravity of her daughter's illness.

Hilary, a Mediterranean beauty, sat holding her son beside Jennifer. She had never been to a seder and I could see the awe on her face as she felt the power of this family.

I, too, was struck by the matriarchy formed by my mother and Aunt Laurie. They were the pillars. Starting from their empty household they had depended on one another yet developed individual strengths. The circle of their lives spread differently but always returned to what was symbolized at this seder table—the two of them, their family, our heritage. That was the feeling there that night. It was a bittersweet picture.

It is children, I decided, who are the lifeline of a family and the heritage parents pass on. Not to have a child is to break the link. Aunt Laurie will abide; she knows that. I can see in her eyes, as she smiles at Jack, Jennifer and Kodie over her Haggadah, that she will go on.

Stanley, who is the son of a cantor, led the ceremony. I could see my aunt keeping a hand or foot or leg on each of her children. Touching, always touching. We went through the entire Haggadah, not a prayer was omitted or uttered without solemn sincerity, no song sung without gaiety.

After dinner, Laurie was tired. Jennifer helped her mother to bed.

"Suzy, would you come in with me?" Laurie asked.

I helped my mother. The sickly-sweet smell of Laurie's medicine clung to the walls and lace curtains of the bedroom. I will never, ever, forget that smell. Mom sat by her sister and began to rub her foot. That big foot of Aunt Laurie's with the crooked toe.

"That's nice," Laurie said. "It makes me feel your closeness."

Jennifer and I left them alone. We knew very well the meaning of that look Laurie gave Jen. "It's our time." We didn't listen by the door as we used to when we were young. This chance for our mothers to be alone was precious; and instinctively, Jen and I knew what was being said.

Laurie removed her jewelry, the lovely necklace, the earring and stud, and pressed them into Suzy's hand. "I want you to have these," she said and leaned over so they could embrace. They held each other a long while. "Here," she said, and gave her sister a small gray felt pouch. "Keep them in here."

Suzy said nothing. Unable to stand up, she reached to Laurie's shoulders. Laurie lay across the bed so they could be in each other's arms. They were quiet, aware that sometimes words destroy feelings. "Suzy," she whispered. "Promise, promise you'll take care of Jennifer and Jack . . . and their children. Be a grandmother to Kodie. Promise."

Suzy buried her head in her sister's neck and nodded; she was choked with emotion and unable to speak a word.

"I know you will. I love you."

"I love you. I love you." They held each other.

Laurie lay back on the pillows and closed her eyes. Smiling. "I'm tired. Stay with me."

Suzy put her hand beneath the blanket and felt her sister's warmth and gently massaged her leg and foot.

"That feels so good, don't stop."

They stayed together just like that.

After a while Jennifer opened the door to check on her mother and I followed her inside. She turned out the light and I helped Mommy up. The walker now seemed heavy for her. I thought Aunt Laurie was asleep. When we reached the door, she murmured, "Thank you for letting me have the seder here. I didn't want to miss it."

Jennifer sat by her mother's bed and held her hand. I heard Aunt Laurie whispering to her as I helped my mother out of the room.

"It's springtime," she said. "Jengi, take me to my house. I want to see my garden. The lilacs should be in bloom and my bleeding hearts, I bet they doubled in size this year. Maybe you and Stanley will prune the perennials with me, and we'll get flowers for the rock garden around the pool. I hope the deer didn't do too much damage, they love the hostas and . . ." Her voice drifted off.

In the bathroom I wiped my mother's tear-streaked face with a cool washcloth. On the perfume tray by the sink top was a large bottle of Chanel No. 5. My mother picked it up and dabbed some on her wrist. She held it to her nose. "This fragrance just isn't the same on me or anyone else as it is on Laurie."

"When she wore it the whole apartment would have her scent. That medicine is foul."

"Oh, Liza, what am I going to do without her?" she sobbed.

I had no answer.

My mother was looking at the photo of herself and her sister wearing wide-brimmed hats. They were arm in arm and laughing. It had been a hot day in late summer, up at Aunt Laurie's house. They were laughing because they had beaten me and Jen at badminton. I know because I had taken the picture.

I knew my mother was remembering as I was; I saw her wipe her eyes. I pressed her hand and we continued to wait, wordlessly, for the phone call from the clinic.

Chapter
11

*W*hen the phone rang I thought I'd have a heart attack.

"Liza Freilicher?"

"Yes."

"Your preg—"—my heart flew up—"—nancy test was negative."

I caught my breath and sobbed. My mother put her arms around me and took my hand.

"Are you okay?" the voice on the phone inquired.

"No. I'm not okay."

"Do you want to talk?"

"No."

The morning after the seder was sunny and warm. Jennifer and Stanley drove Laurie to the house she called home; she had filled it with all her creative energy and meaningful possessions that told the story of her life.

She was too weak to walk and had to be carried up the stairs to her bedroom. Stanley laid her on the great Victorian four-poster bed.

"Jen, I don't want to muss the bed."

Jennifer folded back the crocheted white coverlet and plumped the pillow beneath her mother's head. Laurie surveyed the room: the

glass vitrine displaying small antique treasures she and Jennifer collected together at flea markets or barn auctions, the bureau she
sanded down to the bare mahogany, stained, and polished until it
shone. She could see into the bathroom—the big, claw-footed tub
was under the window where she would lie back in a bubble bath
after gardening all day and watch Jennifer and Jack swim in the
pool below and Stanley feeding carrots to her two burros in the
adjacent corral. It was a room full of loving memories. Memories
of Jennifer and Jack bringing a breakfast tray of pancakes and coffee
upstairs and all of them sitting on the bed to eat. Someone always
dripped syrup on the sheet. They would loll around, tackle the Sunday *Times* crossword puzzle, and then the kids would leave her and
Stanley alone for private times together.

Jennifer covered her mother with a quilt and sat with her long
after she slept.

They stayed at the house. It was May of 1990. Laurie was weaker
each day. The medication no longer kept the pain away, so she was
sedated more heavily. My mother, Greg, and I drove up to the house
almost daily. Stanley and Greg carried my mother upstairs so she
could sit at her sister's bedside. They didn't speak, but Laurie put
out her hand knowing Suzy was there.

One bright morning before Memorial Day, Laurie called to her
daughter.

"Jengi, would you and Stanley help me onto the terrace, I want
to feel the sun and smell the fresh air."

They wrapped her in a blanket and let her rest on the chaise on
the deck outside the bedroom door. Stanley went to the kitchen to
bring tea. Maybe she would drink.

"Mommy, would you like me to do your nails?" Jennifer asked.
"You always like that and I have your color nail polish. It's a new
mauve."

She nodded and Jennifer sat by her side, held her long slender
fingers, and began carefully to file her nails.

"The garden is lovely. I can see the new blooms. Jennifer," she
said, looking at her daughter's bent head. "Jengi . . ."

Jennifer looked up.

"I'm going away soon."

"I know." She was looking into her mother's pale face. For an instant she thought she saw a trace of the old mischief in her eyes. "Mommy, I can't think you will be gone. Don't make me think about it now. Your nails look pretty. Look at them."

Laurie kept her eyes on her daughter's face and said steadily. "We'll make a pact."

Jennifer's eyes brightened. "We'll make a sign so I'll know you are with me, that you'll always be with me."

"What could it be?" Her mother's voice was stronger now. She was enjoying this game, this secret plotting of days gone by. "What could it be? A flash of light? A sudden weird noise? A feather touch on the shoulder? I wonder what powers I'll have."

"Mommy, don't be funny. We need a sign. We have to agree."

"I have to be funny. How else could we have this conversation? What about singing?"

"You can't carry a tune. We'd get mixed up."

Laurie's tone was serious. "What is there, Jengi, that will let you know undoubtedly that I am with you?"

"I'll smell you. It's easy. No one has that special fragrance of Chanel No. 5 when you wear it. I'll know your scent."

"I promise, Jennifer. I'll give you the sign. We have a pact."

Laurie wanted to stay outside surveying the garden, pointing out the new flowers until the afternoon grew cold. Soon, she began to shiver, Jennifer and Stanley carried her to bed for the last time.

THE LOSS AND EMPTINESS inside of me hurt more than any of my imagined pains of childbirth could have hurt. It was the loss of what never existed, the life that might have been mine to bear.

I called David, crying. David, too, began to cry: the thought of all we'd gone through for nothing—all that pain, anger, stress, disappointment, money we had worked hard to earn. Neither of us knew how to proceed.

I couldn't face another in vitro cycle. My brain was spinning.

How could I avoid in vitro and get pregnant? Insemination? Because David's sperm was impacted in his testicles, they were immature and didn't have the power to break into an egg. For this reason insemination could not be done without injecting the sperm into the egg—ICSI. And ICSI couldn't be done without a multiple of harvested eggs. All this information spun in my head repeatedly. There was no way I could become pregnant with David's sperm without another in vitro cycle.

I spoke to David about using the sperm of one of his brothers, or a friend. How weird it would be if I got pregnant with the sperm of a friend or brother-in-law; if our baby was born and we saw the biological father at a party. How would that be? And we'd have to tell the child. No, David and I both agreed, that kind of insemination was not acceptable. Too many compromises.

My mother came up with a ridiculous idea. "Why not go to Spain and visit Rafael?"

"Are you crazy? What are you thinking?"

"You could talk to him about it. Rafael won't be close by; he lives in Spain. Or, you don't have to tell him at all. Birth has been woman's domain throughout history. If you come home pregnant . . . well, you could explain to David that it's his child . . . the blockage miraculously reversed itself. Stranger things have happened."

"Not in today's world, Ma. Not with DNA. Everything is explainable," I retorted, and dismissed the idea.

We laughed, but the idea, crazy as it seemed, remained with me. It didn't upset me morally. The more I thought about it, the saner it became. Rafael was a healthy, clean-living man. There were no serious hereditary illnesses in his family background. His children were healthy and beautiful. Having a child with him would be more meaningful to me than pulling a number out of a hat of sperm donors. It would be an easy way out of another in vitro cycle. "David, the doctor was mistaken, one strong, little sperm pushed its way through." He'd want so badly to believe it. And I thought, for a fleeting moment, he could realize his wish regardless of the cost to my conscience. But our marriage was based on trust. I had to be truthful with my husband.

David listened to the idea of Rafael fathering our child and wasn't completely against it. Poor David. My dear husband took the blow of this suggestion between the eyes and didn't flinch. Perhaps it was callous and unthinking of me. I was racking my brain. I could be comfortable with a pregnancy with Rafael as the donor. If the child could not be of both our genes, at least it would be from me. I thought about it but did nothing.

We had to wait several months after the failed IVF pregnancy before making any decision. David wanted to try another IVF cycle before opting for donor insemination. His argument was that fertilization had at least taken place during the first cycle. I couldn't deny him his chance.

A number of my friends, the women who were my support during IVF at Mount Sinai, had later had success at the Center for Reproductive Medicine and Infertility at New York Hospital—Cornell Medical Center. Even my next-door neighbor, who was now pregnant with twins after having failed for years with IVF, raved about the staff and facility at Cornell.

Cornell is highly rated by the Society of Assisted Reproductive Technology of the American Society for Reproductive Medicine, whose standards are precise and demanding. Of particular interest to me was the embryologist's success rate over the past two years. It was frustrating to think that we could have chosen Cornell earlier; we chose Mount Sinai at the advice of David's urologist, who was affiliated with that hospital, and we felt he was well informed about the technology and staff of the infertility clinic there.

Knowing there was a one-year waiting period to begin treatment at Cornell gave me a breathing time in which to warm up to the idea of beginning IVF again. I felt less pressure than I had before. Also, the infertility clinic at Cornell was separate from the hospital; all the laboratories, treatment areas, and recovery rooms were on-site. No more waiting rooms with blood and sickness.

We put our name on the list and went home, prepared to wait a year.

Chapter

12

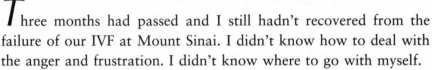

*T*hree months had passed and I still hadn't recovered from the failure of our IVF at Mount Sinai. I didn't know how to deal with the anger and frustration. I didn't know where to go with myself.

I felt I had let David down after he had endured three surgical procedures—the failed reconstruction, the biopsy, and the sperm aspiration. I felt out of control. I had done all I could. I had followed the IVF procedure exactly and had taken care of my health. I spoke warmly, as Jennifer suggested, to the embryos I tried to believe were living inside me. Perhaps it was my doubt that caused the pregnancy to fail. Then, surely, it was my fault.

Patricia told me that many women respond to IVF failure the same way they mourn a death. But it really wasn't like that for me. It wasn't what I experienced when Aunt Laurie passed away. There was no finish, no memorial service, no ashes, no image and memory of times together, no love lost.

There had been a promise of life and now it was a lie. It was a contradiction I could not grasp.

My lack of control over the situation and my emotions frightened me. For the first time I saw something I needed to do and I could not do it. I didn't understand this failure. No one could give a reason for it. The loss of control frightened me so severely that I had moved my focus away from wanting a baby. I no longer envisioned myself holding my baby. The image of David and me with our child, a family, vanished.

IT WAS A SAD TRIP up the Taconic that morning a week after Laurie's death. I drove, Jennifer was quiet in the back next to Kodie, who was asleep in her car seat. Jennifer wanted to pick up some photos and special things of her mother's, anything tangible to keep her mother close. Also, we were bringing a bronze sculpture my mother had made to put in Aunt Laurie's garden to mark the place where her ashes were buried. About an hour out of the city, the road detoured. Teams of men, like ants, were working on new construction. From deep in the earth, the old highway had been blasted apart, the rock sidings flattened and trees downed, to make way for eight lanes of concrete. I slowed and followed the arrows around huge piles of debris. We passed vacated old homesteads, some already devastated skeletons. A few of the families, I imagined, had tried to rebuild; others scattered and moved away, their homes gone. The old stone gas station and local deli where I once stopped were boarded up. Down the road, a shiny new Exxon station was in operation. A McDonald's cranked out food to hungry motorists. The parking lot of a new mall was being landscaped. Dynamite tore apart more than a road; it changed the heart of a town. I turned off at the Poughkeepsie exit and drove through the familiar countryside.

"Do you know how much I wanted to go with her?" Jennifer's voice was flat, barely audible from the backseat. "I never gave up; I thought we would beat it. I didn't want her to go alone. I wish I were with her. I wish I were with her," she sobbed. "There is no purpose for me now."

I reached my hand behind me to touch her head, which she had leaned forward against the window. "Jen, turn around. Look at your daughter. Look at Kodie. She's your life now."

"I'm going to stay up here at the house. I can't go back to Chicago with Stephen."

"Jen, it's been two weeks. It takes a long time to begin to heal. You have to let him help you."

"I don't want to go back. Here is the only place I can be close to her. She's here. She's in every inch of this house. I hate Stephen. He tries to take my mother's place. I hate him for trying."

"Don't be angry with him because he's who you're left with. He's trying to be everything to you. He can't be, I know, but, Jen, let him comfort you."

"I don't want him or anyone close to me. He can't fulfill me the way my mother did. He can't do anything for me."

"He's suffering, too, you know. He loved Laurie."

"He doesn't know the first thing about it." She moved her head away from my hand in anger.

We came to the big oak tree and turned down the drive. My body ached to be coming to the home where Aunt Laurie used to run out of the front door in greeting. Jennifer was holding Kodie and crying as we stopped in front of the empty house.

I stayed for two days with Jen and Kodie. We put the sculpture in the garden. It is a nude torso of a young woman with firm breasts and an arched back, sitting back on her heels.

Years ago, Laurie had said, "I wish you'd give me that," and my mother laughed. It was her masterpiece and she wanted to live with it. My mother knew her sister would understand. She acknowledged that the love between them was unconditional and thus Laurie was the easiest person to say no to.

"I wish I had given it to her then," my mother said when we loaded the sculpture into the car early that morning.

Jennifer went through the motions of shopping, preparing meals and trying to eat, but they were just motions. When I sensed that she wanted to be alone, I left.

After a week, Jennifer and Kodie flew back to Chicago. Stephen picked them up at the airport. I was worried about Jen. She seemed to be in a bubble, floating, not alert to what was happening, not participating.

Jennifer and Stephen lived in a large house in Lake Forest, an elite suburb. Jennifer planned to raise her family there. It was her dream—one husband, one home, no moving for her children. It represented financial and emotional stability. Her entire concentration was on making that dream come true. A secure home for Kodie. She was the center of her life. Jennifer kept her husband away physically, mentally, and emotionally. All that existed was Dakota.

Some couples, Patricia said, grow closer when they suffer a mutual loss. They are bonded by the need to decide whether to undergo the rigors of another assisted pregnancy. Other couples, she said, separate themselves from each other emotionally, feeling that what each endured he or she endured alone.

David and I fell into neither category. We were united by desire. But we internalized the disappointment and that set us apart. I was angry with David because he didn't express the same burning rage as I did. He tolerated my pessimism but would not be defeated.

What was most frustrating was that it seemed that we had what it took; Dr. Blake of Mount Sinai was unable to explain our failure. "Your eggs were mature and bountiful. David's sperm was viable. You had excellent cell division and six healthy embryos were implanted."

We called her constantly, hoping that she had found an answer, a missing puzzle piece that would reveal what we could do differently if we decided to try ICSI all over again.

In January of 1995, three months after our Mount Sinai IVF failure, I was at home at nine in the morning folding laundry when the phone rang and Dr. Blake introduced me to the Immunological Factor. She had just returned from a seminar where this theory had been hotly discussed.

"It's possible," she explained, "that the antibodies in your blood, Liza, identified the transferred embryos as invaders and were arming up to fight them off."

The doctor explained that antibodies play a role in miscarriage. Women who have recurrent miscarriages tend to have high levels of antisperm antibodies. Some doctors believe these antisperm antibodies may interfere with normal embryo development. Also, women who develop antibodies against sperm may also develop other immune-system responses that may be involved in causing miscarriages.

She concluded by saying, "Liza, I think you should contact the genetic IVF institute in Fairfax, Virginia. They specialize in immunology."

There was relief in receiving Dr. Blake's call. Finally, we had been given a possible cause for the failure of the IVF cycle. David and I agreed that our problem was different from those of my cohorts who had found success with IVF. All the doctors and technicians at Mount Sinai were of the opinion that the immunity factor was key to our IVF failure and that not to pursue it with the specialists in that field at Fairfax would be negligent on our part.

I had one final question for Dr. Blake. "Is the immunological factor a common cause of infertility?" I asked, hoping the cure was much practiced and something I could depend on.

"I can't say it's common. It is just one of the possibilities in the major problem of infertility."

My emotional stability was so very fragile that the slightest hope or fear could push me into ecstasy or despair. Having been told that the failure of the IVF was probably linked to the immunological immunity factor, a fact that could be acted upon, somehow freed me from guilt. I made the decision to do another IVF cycle at Fairfax. I was heading in a forward direction and that gave me the sense that I was gaining control over my infertility problem.

Chapter

13

*F*airfax would not accept us without a preliminary consultation. David and I took a train to Washington, D.C. The day was gray.

We took a cab for the half-hour drive from the Capitol to the clinic. The waiting room was decorated with large built-in fish tanks, which made the environment very peaceful. A positive sign. I liked the idea that this was a self-contained unit treating only infertility. Finally, no more sharing a waiting room with pregnant women, whose success always seemed to increase my sense of failure.

First we met with the urologist. He seemed insightful and modestly optimistic. He said under no conditions would he begin treatment prior to six months after David's last surgical procedure. This disappointed us. I wanted to start immediately. Waiting only gave me time to worry and develop cold feet, which meant, inevitably, that I would have to go through the agony of making a decision all over again.

An hour later we met with Dr. Willa Holbrook. She was supposed to be more knowledgeable about the use of blood thinners and the immunological factor than the staff at Mount Sinai.

"It is no mystery," she said, trying to put the medical data in our chart in lay terms. "Liza, your eggs are healthy. David's sperm, though immature, did fertilize the eggs, you had good cell division. We have to look elsewhere for the problem. Liza's blood condition jumps out as the source. She must continue on blood thinners if she is to undergo another IVF cycle, as those medications tend to thicken the blood and would aggravate her blood-clotting condition, putting her health in jeopardy. However, Liza, that blood condition is separate from the reason the embryos were rejected from your uterus. The clues presented here lead me to believe the reason for your failure to hold these embryos was the immunological factor. It is possible your blood built up antibodies against these embryos, as invaders, and forced them out. Do I make myself clear?"

David and I nodded. She sounded like Sherlock Holmes.

Dr. Holbrook continued. "Therefore we could try to use a new medicine to keep these antibodies from forming. It is speculation, I want to emphasize that, but in my opinion the best approach. I must tell you again, keep in mind these treatments are experimental."

She suggested administering antibodies through the use of a permanent pump installed as an IV that dripped into my body twenty-four hours a day. I would have to live ten months of my life walking around with an intravenous apparatus—the one month of IVF before the eggs are harvested and fertilized and nine months of pregnancy. I refused.

Aunt Laurie had worn such an apparatus to administer the experimental medicine that didn't save her life. Just to remember the smell of the stuff still nauseated me.

And then, of course, there was the risk of HIV and other diseases, because the antibody medications are made from donated blood. Dr. Holbrook thought I would eventually come around and change my mind. She was wrong. I was certain of that.

David and I had many questions, but suddenly the doctor was in a hurry and cut us short. After fifteen minutes, we were being ushered out. We had made the trip, taken time from work, lived the full day around infertility again. They insisted that we meet in person, that a phone consultation would not do. And now they wanted six hundred dollars. Even David, who is usually unruffled, was angry.

We considered doing an IVF cycle in three months but refused Dr. Holbrook's suggestion of administering the antibodies intravenously. The risk of HIV was substantial, plus the uncertainty and experimental status of the treatment, plus living with intravenous for ten months—all this was unacceptable to David and me. Dr. Holbrook remained expressionless as we explained our decision, then said that the immunological treatment was just another approach and didn't preclude a second attempt at IVF.

I sensed that Dr. Holbrook didn't like me. Was I becoming paranoid? I hated all doctors and was desperate for something to give me courage.

IN OCTOBER 1990, five months after Aunt Laurie's death, I flew out to Chicago to spend Jennifer's birthday with her. She told me she was trying to get pregnant. I was happy. I thought it was a sign that she was relating better to Stephen and told her so.

"No," she said. "I want another baby because I don't want Dakota to be alone and have to take care of me. When Mommy had me she was very young, scared, and lonely. For a long time, we only had each other. I was the center of her universe and she was the center of mine. We had no boundaries. I don't want Dakota to have the same neediness."

Jen liked to cook. She had a whole bookcase of cookbooks in her state-of-the-art kitchen. We made chocolate-chip cookies. I scraped the bowl and licked the batter while she dropped the last spoonful onto the greased cookie sheet and spoke freely to me.

"Kodie will have self-esteem, and be able to satisfy her own needs, not mine. You know, Lollipop, I created her totally out of selfishness. I created her to save myself from my mother's death, so I wouldn't be alone."

A few weeks later, when Thanksgiving arrived, we decided to keep family tradition alive. Jennifer came to New York and went directly to her mother's country house with Stephen, Kodie, and Stephen's daughters, Alexis and Devan. I drove up early on Thursday morning with Mommy and Erica so we could help Jen cook. Greg met us with Max and Stuart. Stanley was there when we arrived. Jack would arrive in time for dinner.

The house was bustling. Stephen carried Mommy up the hill and into the kitchen. I brought in some groceries and started to mash the yams for sweet-potato pie. Jen was stuffing a colossal turkey. "Stanley," she called, "where's Mommy's porcelain bread box?"

He was in the living room, piling logs into the fireplace. "I brought it to New York, to my apartment."

Jennifer stopped working. She wiped her hands on her apron and looked at the ceiling. "That bread box, I was with her when she bought it at the flea market. It belongs here. You can't move it."

A log thumped down loudly, then another. "I like seeing it in the morning; this is my house, Jennifer, what's in it is mine."

She didn't move. Then she picked up the spoon and continued stuffing the bird. Her voice was low and controlled when she spoke. "This is my mother's house."

Stanley didn't answer, and remained silent and withdrawn for the rest of the evening.

I looked at Jennifer surrounded by family. Kodie was playing with Stephen's older daughters; Greg's son, Stuart, was creeping about the floor. All these children. Jennifer was in the midst of the chaos, the sturdy pillar of unity and strength. I felt like an outsider. I looked at my mother at the table cutting vegetables. She no longer seemed like a bulwark. And I saw the hole my aunt Laurie's absence made in the picture of my family. Both Jennifer and I had been raised by our mothers, Jennifer, because of early divorce, and I because my father was consumed by his work and hobbies. We regarded our mothers as the fountainhead of our physical, emotional, and material well-being. In many confidences to each other, from childhood to this day, we admired the centrality of women in our family and wished to emulate our mothers.

I asked Jennifer if she felt this had become a burden, and was surprised at her answer.

She told me she was hardly aware of it, that assuming her mother's role was a natural evolution, a role she played with joy and pride. "Liza, part of this legacy is for you to stand beside me with your own children," she said.

Another concern about the Virginia clinic was that we would have to stay there for five weeks. We had to be there for preliminary blood tests even before the first injection, and remain for daily blood tests and medication monitoring during the period of egg retrieval, ICSI, fertilization, and transfer of the embryos. It was a long time for working people to put a stop to their lives. We would have to stay in a hotel, and rent a car, all of which added to the expense.

Fortunately, Dr. Holbrook gave us the decisive option of remaining in New York and working with a private doctor who would send the daily blood reports and sonograms. The doctors in Fairfax would thus be able to monitor the medications. She referred us to Dr. Michael Owins, who had originally been at Mount Sinai. He agreed to work along with the Fairfax doctors during the preliminary tests, which would shorten our stay in Virginia from five weeks to two.

Everything made sense: the specialists in the immunity factor would be watching my blood, and I would only be seen by Dr. Owins in New York and then be treated at the Fairfax Clinic, which was solely for infertility, and therefore, to my mind, insulated from sickness and death. David and I agreed with optimism.

However, I had to supply the Fairfax Clinic with donor sperm. It was a precaution, in case, when the time came, they couldn't obtain mature sperm from David to fertilize the harvested eggs. David was convinced he could produce good sperm; he had done so before. Nonetheless, we arranged to transport the original frozen donor sperm #2047 in a rented nitrogen-oxide tank to the Fairfax Clinic.

Dr. Owins did the sonograms and took my blood each morning. Every day I had to arrange to have the specimens sent to the clinic in Fairfax by Federal Express in special blood transportation packages supplied by the blood laboratory. Fairfax insisted on having the blood analyzed in their laboratories by the same technicians who would do my blood workup when I arrived. They were the experts and they had the responsibility of prescribing medicines; they, too, wanted successful live births for their own records. Experimentation in and treatment of infertility had become a competitive business, which in the long run was beneficial to the patient.

My entire day became consumed by the blood tests and getting the blood to Virginia on time for the lab to analyze and determine daily medication dosages. As before, I had to track down the medications, and resorted to stalking the pharmacies on my earlier list.

One weekday, Federal Express missed the blood pickup. It was a crucial blood test to determine whether I should begin the Pergonal injections that night; therefore, my blood had to be in the Fairfax lab early that afternoon.

Pergonal is the hormone used to stimulate ovulation so that multiple fertilized eggs will be available at the time of retrieval. It is administered between the first and fifth day of the cycle depending on the blood levels, which have been checked daily to indicate when the largest number of follicles can be recruited and the eggs inside those follicles are developing well.

I called David, desperately seeking a way to get the blood to Virginia. David's assistant, Madaline, overheard us speaking.

"I'm from Washington," she said. "I can deliver it for you and I'll visit my parents."

So many people were anxious to help us, if only I kept myself open to notice. Being open to people was always difficult to me. That David's and my infertility problem was common knowledge made me uncomfortable. David discussed it with his close associates. For him, friends were as close as family. It seemed our life was fair game for conversation and it made me feel invaded even if these people meant to be encouraging. "A baby should be created out of love and now ours will be a scientific process," I cried to Jennifer.

"No," Jennifer told me emphatically. "When you have a baby it will be out of the greatest love, and science will make it all possible. IVF is about having a baby, without it your quest would be hopeless."

Madaline took a plane that afternoon in the midst of a snowstorm. She arrived at the Fairfax Clinic just in time for them to analyze the blood specimen. I was grateful. Jennifer had made me see clearly, and like a pendulum I swung to optimism.

Chapter

14

Our trip to Virginia was fast approaching. I called our friends Carol and Randy, who lived in Washington, D.C. I thought they might recommend a hotel and some places for us to go for day trips. We planned to use the free time away from the clinic as a vacation.

Carol had known David since they played ring-a-levio on the Yonkers Elementary School playground. I had known her only briefly, from our wedding and a few in-town-for-the-day dinner engagements. Carol insisted I stay with them, but I declined. I knew I would not want company with Lupron coursing through my veins. I feared the hateful creature I became with that medication.

"Liza," Carol said, her voice quiet but steady, "I went through four years of infertility. I finally gave up treatment—that's when we adopted Jake. I know what you're going through. I think you'll be more comfortable here in our home, rather than an impersonal hotel. We'll cook, you won't have to dress and look for restaurants each meal. Randy and I are out at work all day, so you'll have plenty of privacy and quiet time."

I had known Jake was adopted but never discussed the circumstances with Carol. This goes back to my code of silence concerning personal matters. I hoped that spending this time with Carol, Randy, and Jake as a family would help me become more acquainted with adoption, even though I prayed we would not have to face it. Carol was offering more than a place to stay; she was willing to share my doubts and fears and reveal her own struggles. I had promised myself and Jennifer to accept whatever help was offered and so I accepted Carol's invitation.

We drove down to Washington so we wouldn't have to rent a car. Carol had set up her den as a bedroom.

The walls were pine-paneled. There was a floral-print convertible sofa bed and a grass-colored carpet. It was airy and bright. A television sat on a bookshelf packed with paperbacks.

"Looks like you won't be bored while I sleep," I joked with David. He is an avid reader.

"Or I could play those video games" he said, indicating Jake's stack beside the TV.

"That's kids today," I said. "Maybe Jake can teach me. I'll have plenty of time."

"I'll teach you," the six-year-old announced, smiling up at me. He was fair-haired and blue-eyed, unlike Carol and Randy, though I recognized Carol in his impish sense of humor and Randy in his straightforwardness and stance. Jake may have been adopted, but he was clearly their son.

Carol showed us an empty closet and the bathroom. She looked pleased that we found the room pleasant.

Monday morning we checked into the Fairfax Clinic. I went for all the tests and continued my medications. As no distinctive antibodies appeared in my blood and I had declined the intravenous drip, this IVF was, in effect, the same procedure as I had undergone at Mount Sinai, except in a more congenial atmosphere. Dr. Holbrook and the technicians were upbeat saying. "Each time a couple has sex, they don't conceive. It's the same with IVF. There are no guarantees, no matter how ideal the conditions appear. You must give IVF another try."

It was better to be out of New York City and have new places to discover. We managed to take an afternoon trip to the Air and Space Museum. It was an ordinary thing to do, but for us it was special.

I was struck by the speed of technological advances as I traced the path that led from the plane that flew at Kitty Hawk to the mooncraft and present-day missiles. One hundred years ago we were in the dark ages and now outer space was a crossable frontier. I saw how if not for scientific advancement, many women would still be dying in childbirth. The true beauty of this museum is the testimony it provides of man's persistence, and through my treatments, I was part of this history. I felt better than I had in a long time.

By my second week on Lupron, my emotions and moods were turbulent. As the feeling of doom became more intense, I told myself this IVF cycle would not work. David and I began to argue.

From the sonograms the doctors saw that my ovaries were not responding as well as they had during the last cycle. There were just a few follicles. They had no explanation for it. They didn't rule out stress as a factor. Stress, they said, can reduce the output of hormones that stimulate the pituitary gland to send signals to the ovaries.

I had no control over the stress. Just trying to control it made it worse. David suggested another museum as a diversion. I felt sluggish and had neither the energy nor the patience for a leisurely walk. What I wanted to do more than anything was visit an Arabian horse farm south of D.C. that I had read about. David agreed.

It was a two-hour drive. David and I were absorbed in our own thoughts. There was no need to talk. It was serene just to be moving freely through the green rolling hills of Virginia and letting my mind wander away from IVF. I wanted to visit the Arabian horse farm because I had always been awed by the majesty of these animals. I had even thought about owning one.

A stable hand was waiting for us when we arrived at the office. In one barn there were only stallions, some champion studs. Other barns had geldings, horses at different stages of schooling, with ribbons and photos hanging above their stalls. I liked the one-year-olds. Their barn was filled with the sweet, warm scent of young horseflesh and hay I remembered from my childhood. The yearlings were so eager. They came up to me and nuzzled my hand. Arabians are close-coupled; the distance between their front and rear legs is shorter than in the hunters that I used to ride. These young Arabians were gentle and flirtatious, not nervous and skittish, with their velvety noses that sloped upward instead of being severely straight, their long and flowing manes, and their tied up tails to keep them from dragging in the sawdust. One horse in particular enchanted me. He was gray, and I was told he would become much whiter as he matured. His eyes were soft and for a crazy moment I longed to bring him home. I could forget all about this childbearing agony and have this sweet, exquisite animal to train and care for. Childbearing? I thought suddenly. If I could feel this way for a horse after ten minutes, what would I feel toward an adopted baby? Perhaps I would love a child entrusted to me to protect, guide, and care for. He would be my child and I would love him unconditionally.

I was silent on the way back. For the first time, I was thinking a bit more positively about adoption. It may be I was already rationalizing the failure that threatened.

Your ovaries are not responding as expected.

Was I trying to protect myself from the disappointment that followed the Mount Sinai IVF?

In just an afternoon, I was feeling more openminded about adoption. I thought of Carol going about her life with her adopted son and how it was a brave thing to do and had brought happiness instead of pain.

I had been seeking happiness myself in much the same way when I first met David.

I MET DAVID in 1991 a few months after Ben and I broke up. I was fed up with meaningless dates and dead-end relationships. I was anxious to meet a man I could consider spending the rest of my life with. I was thinking of marriage and then of children. I was thinking of taking my rightful place beside Jennifer in the legacy passed to us by my mother and Aunt Laurie.

Christmas and New Year's were at last over. The restaurant had been very busy since Thanksgiving, with corporate parties and tourists. I never got to bed before two A.M. Call me the perennial Scrooge, but I was pleased to take down the twinkling lights and bows over the bar.

My spirits were high even when the hostess called me aside at dinner to say the toilet in the ladies' room was stopped up; I was an expert at this. I picked up the plunger and went into combat. I came out victorious, the plunger hidden behind me, when she signaled to me and pointed to the bar, mouthing, "Your date."

I had completely forgotten that David Freilicher, a friend of a friend, had called that morning. He asked me to go out with him for a drink. I wouldn't take time away from work for someone I didn't know. We decided to meet at the restaurant.

"I'll check you out," he said jokingly.

"And I'll check *you* out. Nine o'clock at the bar . . . that good?"

"Fine. We'll decide then if it's worth having dinner another night."

Oh my gosh! And now he'd seen me with a plunger.

He came over to greet me. He was smiling, a mischievous smile, and had blue eyes, a good build. Cute. "So, the restaurant business is really glamorous, isn't it?"

"As glamorous as you can make it," I retorted coyly.

"Good job," he said, taking the plunger from me, opening the bathroom door, and putting it inside, relieving my embarrassment.

Immediately it was a relaxed encounter. We had shared a comical experience and from then on were talking about what we enjoyed and found humorous instead of the usual mundane question-and-answer period of dates.

I ordered a vodka gimlet and we made jokes about fancy restaurateurs. We made a date for brunch, Sunday, at the Carlyle Hotel. It was the first date I'd looked forward to in a long time. David and I clicked.

To David and me, hotel dining rooms have a special appeal. The Carlyle, an oasis of civility, is one of our favorites.

After brunch, we went to the Museum of Modern Art and passed through the antiques show at the Sixty-sixth Street Armory on Park Avenue. Then we went to the movies. We didn't want the date to end.

That evening, David came home with me and I changed into a black scoop-neck sweater and black slacks. I loaned him a unisex black turtleneck sweater and the two of us went out, laughing, as sleek panthers. We had dinner at Fujiyama Mama, a trendy Japanese restaurant, and sampled from a large array of sushi.

David was going to Florida to visit his parents early the next morning, and I was about to embark on a much-needed weeklong sailing trip with Greg, Maxine, and the baby. My flight with Greg to Miami left at noon.

The boat was luxurious. I shared a cabin with Stuart because I didn't want him to be alone. Greg and Max had the large aft cabin. There were two baths with showers. The salon was paneled with rich mahogany. The sofas were plush, but we spent all our time outside on the spacious rear deck. A barbecue grill hung over the rail, and there we cooked all the fresh seafood we bought from the local fisherman. I was brown, slippery with suntan oil, and relaxed. My body was strong from swimming. I enjoyed snorkeling; looking down at the reefs made me feel as if I were weightless and flying. At night we'd moor out in different coves of the Bahamas Out Islands and listen to reggae music from the beach bars while sipping fruit-and-rum drinks Greg concocted. David called me every night. We were already close, just from our single marathon date. We made a date to celebrate my return.

The next morning we set out early from Nassau to the Keys to return the rented boat. The sky was ominously overcast. It was a two-hour trip to the coast, where we planned to stop for lunch, and then another hour to the marina in Key Largo to return the boat. After that, it would be an hour-and-a-half car drive to the airport in Miami. The seas were high and the boat rose and fell into the deep troughs the waves made. I held on to Stuart, who was crying, sick to his stomach and fighting to pull off his life vest. I rocked him in my arms. At last he fell asleep.

It started to rain. The wind was whipping up whitecaps. Greg was on the bridge with Max. I wanted to take Stuart below to lay him on the bed. When I stood up my left foot felt as if it were numb, all pins and needles. I stomped on it to get the blood flowing, but instead of going away, the numbness crept up the left side of my body. I couldn't lift my left arm or leg. My head ached; I was nauseous and trembling with icy chills and fear. I didn't know what to do. Greg was maneuvering the boat. When the pins and needles went up to my chest and face, I panicked. I didn't know what was happening and thought I would die at any moment. I called Max to come and take Stuart. She carried him below and went to the bridge to tell Greg that I was ill.

"I'm radioing an ambulance to meet us at the dock," he hollered down over the noise of the engine and wind. "I'm sure it's nothing, but I'm calling the ambulance anyway." He had noticed that my lips were blue. "Stay calm, La, sit down. You're white."

The Emergency Medical Service met us at the boat dock. There were two young paramedics. They asked my age.

"Twenty-nine." I told them my symptoms.

They looked bewildered. "If you were eighty years old, I'd say you had had a stroke," said one.

"We're going to take you to the hospital."

I wasn't going anywhere with those two kids. I called my doctor in New York and told him what had transpired. We spent thirty minutes talking and by then the strength was slowly returning to my arm.

"Wait ten minutes and call me back. I'm right here by the phone. See how you feel in ten minutes," Dr. Goldstein said.

When I called him back, I was feeling a little better. The numbness was subsiding and my arm and leg were stronger. Not normal, but stronger.

"Don't miss your plane. Go right to the emergency room at Roosevelt Hospital. I'll meet you there."

Later, at La Guardia Airport, while Greg went for the car, I called my mother. She said she'd have my father meet me at the hospital. Greg and I took a cab into the city together. Max drove their car home with Stuart.

I had asked Greg to call David and tell him what happened and that I wouldn't be home for our date. David didn't hesitate to come to the hospital. I was surprised and embarrassed, but happy to see he was there waiting for me.

Dr. Goldstein did blood and urine tests and checked my reflexes. He wanted me to stay overnight for observation, he said.

"Observation of what?" I asked, still feeling weak, but I had regained sensation in my left side.

"Liza, I think this is nothing. Perhaps a drop in your blood pressure, also stress, but I would be at fault not to pursue it. I want to reassure myself by scheduling an MRI of your head."

The words sent terror throughout my body. I envisioned my sister, Erica. Was her condition genetic? What was going to befall me now that I was on the brink of happiness with David? Was it my grandmother's omen over again? *Suzy, you are the luckiest girl* . . .

I refused to stay in the hospital. David took me home. He called me once he got back to his apartment to make sure I was okay.

The next morning I returned to the hospital for an MRI of my head, which showed scar tissue.

"Liza, you've had a mini-stroke. The medical term is TIA—transient ischemic attack. We have to find out what caused it."

In the weeks that followed, I went to a hematologist, a cardiologist, and a neurologist. The hematologist discovered that I had a blood-clotting disorder and suggested I go off birth-control pills because they thicken the blood, and that, combined with this blood disorder, could have been the cause of the TIA. I was put on aspirin therapy. "One aspirin tablet daily is a mild treatment to keep the blood thin. I don't expect another recurrence."

I was scared. Every time my foot fell asleep, I would panic that I was having a stroke. I tried to hide this fear from everyone; I didn't want to make a big deal out of it.

David never left me without planning our next date. He never played games, always called when he said he would. Soon we were a couple. It was as if each of us had recognized in the other a soul mate. I knew he was dependable and wouldn't falter. We balanced each other. David is more structured and conservative than I am. I dive into a project wholeheartedly and impulsively. I see the end, then I work until I get there. David reads the map. I go by instinct, but we arrive at the same place. After one year of dating, David and I decided to rent an apartment together.

I didn't have another mini-stroke and tried to forget about it, except that I took an aspirin with my vitamins each morning. And David was there to make sure I did. It was great knowing he would be home when I returned from the long nights at the restaurant.

I loved feeling his body next to me when we slept. I was safe. And when he left for work in the morning, I enjoyed knowing he thought of me and cared about me during the day and that we'd be together again after work.

We set the day for our wedding, a Saturday in May, one and a half years after that marathon date.

Jennifer could not come to New York before the day of the wedding. She was facing another calamity in her life, one she told me she should have seen coming. She had been immersed in Dakota and in her house and so was unaware of the changing atmosphere in the business world. The media companies were downsizing. People like her husband, Stephen Scheu, who had worked for one company for seventeen years, suddenly found themselves unemployed. He was given a full year's salary as severance pay. That, he assured her, bought time and he would find a job. Jennifer refused to believe her house was in jeopardy.

I was concerned about my cousin. She was acting out of character. She had always been a take-charge woman. Now it appeared she was turning inward. She refused to see the reality of her situation and didn't want to discuss it even with me. It was as if she found refuge within herself, where she said her mother was.

On my wedding day, my bridal party was given a suite in the Fifth Avenue mansion that was the Metropolitan Club, where we were married. The flower-bedecked dressing room accommodated me, my mother, Maxine, and Jennifer, who was my matron of honor. I arrived early that morning. I wanted to spend the whole day there. It was like being in another era, an age of chivalry that I envied. From the window I looked down on horse-drawn carriages and the golden fountain in front of the Plaza Hotel, where Mr. and Mrs. David Freilicher would spend their wedding night before flying off to the south of France for a honeymoon.

Jennifer helped me put on my makeup. Mom took pictures of us getting dressed and we had a light snack sent up. The ceremony was to start at 7:30 P.M.

"Jen, you look especially bright today."

"I'm happy for you, Lollipop, and"—she stepped into her pencil-straight strapless gown, turned, and let Mommy zip her up—"I'm pregnant!" She was grinning. Jennifer saw her second pregnancy as an emotional panacea.

I was pulling up my bridal garter and stopped at the knee. "Jen, another child *now*, with Stephen's job situation?"

"Well, we stopped trying after he got fired, but it just happened. I'm so excited." She smiled the naughty grin of the Cheshire cat.

I was thrilled for her; there was life back in her voice.

"So, we have two wonderful occasions to celebrate," my mother concluded. "Come on, my girls, let's start now." She popped the cork on a bottle of Dom Pérignon that was cooling in the ice bucket beside the little gray pouch of jewelry she had given me to wear for my wedding.

My descent down the magnificent staircase was as spectacular as I'd always dreamed. Stuart was an impish ring bearer and Kodie the angelic flower girl. Greg was the number-one usher along with David's two brothers. David's closest friend, James, was best man. Erica and Max were bridesmaids.

This time my mother was helped to the chupa by her boyfriend, Joe. They had met four years earlier at the Sculpture Studio and had been together since.

My father gave the bride away to the relieved groom. It seemed to David that we had been arranging this gala for an eternity.

I now perceived this impending IVF failure as an emotional holocaust.

I didn't want to go through retrieval, now that I was leaning toward adoption. If the eggs were not responsive, it meant I was inadequate. I didn't want to face that. Adoption was the way to go. When I told this to the doctor, she wouldn't listen.

"Liza, we just need one egg. One egg."

On the day of retrieval, two days after our trip to the horse farm, the urologist told us he had good specimen from David. Dr. Holbrook harvested five eggs from my uterus, which were immediately given to the embryologist for ICSI.

Dr. Holbrook came into the recovery room to tell us that we could leave. She was a maddeningly pedantic woman who offered no moral support when we voiced our worries. "Time will tell," she said. "We have three days to watch the cell division. Each day will show more of the fertilization results."

Once again there was nothing to do but go home and leave our future in a petri dish with the embryologist.

Chapter

15

*W*e went back to the room that Carol had fixed for us. There were flowers on the table beside the convertible sofa. It was Carol's way of respecting my privacy and showing her understanding without a word. I had underestimated Carol, as I had many people, and found solace in remembering Jennifer's words about people truly wanting to help and how not everything could be achieved alone.

I put my hands on my swollen belly. David was setting up the tray to give me my next shot of progesterone—that slow, thick serum caused more bloating and was very painful. There were tears in my eyes; soon I would be crying. David didn't look at me. He filled the syringe with the progesterone, which, along with estrogen, directs the lining of the uterus to produce a blanket of blood cells and the glands to secrete the nourishment the fertilized eggs need to survive. I had read so many fertility guidebooks I could write a usage manual for these drugs myself.

I watched David mechanically doing what had to be done, with no more outward anxiety than he'd have brushing his teeth. Even the surgical procedure for sperm aspiration had not ruffled him. He seemed to have put all emotion aside. Keep it simple; get the job done—that was David's attitude. I, on the other hand, could not set my emotions aside. Didn't David understand what was happening? We had small, inadequate eggs. Nothing was going happen. There was no escape.

I felt as if I were choking. I was closed in; there was nothing beyond this endless cycle of IVF. I went into the bathroom.

"Liza?" David called. "Are you all right?"

I closed the door and turned on the water in the sink full force to drown the sound of my sobs. I was weak from crying and I slid down to my knees on the bathroom floor.

David opened the door. He sat down on the cold tile floor and held me.

I put my arms around him. It had been so long since we had been in each other's arms. We were afraid to touch one another. I needed very much to know the closeness that only feeling, smelling, and touching brings.

"I'm so lonesome, David. Help me. I can't hold on to myself."

He cradled me there in that dark little bathroom, and rocked me and let me cry. He rubbed my head and wiped my tears and I felt protected; the frightened feeling ebbed with my tears. I closed my eyes and pressed my body to him until my arms ached. We rocked back and forth. I felt better, stronger. He picked me up and carried me to the sofa.

"I love you, Liza," my husband said. He was sobbing. I held him, and wiped his eyes with kisses. I had been so absorbed in myself I hadn't considered that David, too, was suffering.

Through the open door of the bathroom I saw the vase of flowers on the table.

"I'm ready for the injection," I said. I didn't cry. I had no more tears. It seemed trivial to cry for a pain that would pass.

David and I wanted to do something for Carol and Randy to acknowledge their generosity. David found some furniture polish and went into the living room. An hour later I felt strong enough to get up. The house was gleaming. Even the tarnished candlesticks in the center of the dining-room table shone. I went into the kitchen and made tollhouse cookies from Jennifer's recipe, and let David sample a few as they came from the oven.

I could hear Jennifer's voice telling me, "Liza, I have a theory. If you share with others, you lessen your load." She was right; making these cookies and fixing the house was not all for Carol and Randy. It was giving me pleasure. It was getting up and moving away from my troubles. Both David and I were smiling.

Carol was thrilled to see the transformation when she came home, and this made me happy. You have to give to get, I thought more and more often.

The next day I brought a tin of cookies for the staff at the hospital. They told us they had done assisted hatching. The embryologist said cell division was not looking strong. As the day of the transfer neared, I was pessimistic.

"One good egg, Liza. We just need one good egg."

On the day before the transfer, we went to the hospital with low expectations. Dr. Holbrook told us we had four embryos but with low cell division. She explained, "Ideally by twenty-four hours after fertilization, the sperm and egg should become a two-celled pre-embryo. By forty-eight hours that pre-embryo should have four cells and by seventy-two hours after fertilization there should be eight cells. Without healthy cell division, we do not have a healthy embryo to transfer. An embryo without good cell division will not adhere to the uterus."

I started to cry. I hoped some miracle would occur overnight and there would be a more favorable result. "Is it even worth doing the transfer?' I asked.

"What have you got to lose? You should definitely transfer. You never know."

Sure. It was easy for her to say. If the transfer failed, it would be heart-wrenching. My expression must have revealed my thoughts.

"It's up to you. I'll leave the room while you decide."

She seemed to have no patience with emotion. She was there to perform a service which we had chosen to have done and were paying her to do. Now I was confronting her with raw feelings, putting obstacles in her way. If she became emotional with each patient, she would be useless in her job. I could understand her position, but I didn't forgive her. In my opinion, empathizing with patients and trying to help them through the difficult times was part of a doctor's job.

David, true to himself, was not deterred. "Liza, let's just do it. We're so close."

The following morning we did the transfer. I was not put to sleep. The embryos were inserted into my uterus using a catheter, as had been done at Mount Sinai. There was some pain. I watched on the sonogram screen. This time I looked on in a clinically dispassionate way. I was a veteran, and I wasn't a fool. I had known disappointment. Those images did not promise life. They promised nothing. The whole enterprise was futile.

The procedure was over in twenty minutes. An hour later, they said I could go home, rest for two days, and then I would be fine to drive back to New York. I lay in bed for two days while David was out to the grocery store or video store. It was quiet, except when Jake was playing his monotonous video games. When we were ready to depart for New York, Randy brought our luggage to the car. I was walking slowly, afraid any sudden movement might dislodge an embryo. I thought that the next time we spoke to Randy and Carol, we'd know whether we were pregnant. Our stay at their home had brought David closer to his old friends and I got to know them as friends as well. Carol kept reiterating how she loved her son. She said adoption was a blessing and that she felt Jake was as much hers as if he'd come from her own body.

I believed Carol, but there was an embryo of our own now inside me, and I was desperate to believe that David and I were pregnant with our biological child.

Carol kissed me good-bye. "Liza, we loved having you with us. I'm glad you got to know Jake."

Randy hugged me warmly. He hugged David also and patted his back the way men do to show their affection.

David drove home slowly. We counted the minutes of the two endless, miserable weeks before the pregnancy test. I didn't believe I was pregnant because of the embryo quality.

Jennifer and I spoke often. When I told her of my doubts, she said, "Hold on, will it to happen." It was the same advice she had given me the first time. When I tried to discuss adoption, she closed the door on the subject. "You haven't come to that."

My mother replied as Jennifer had. "Liza, you have done so much; don't give up. I haven't," and she spent time with me at my apartment.

I had endured the agony of waiting before, but this time it was worse. I felt as if I was in an endless tunnel. I didn't sleep. I was tired. I forced myself to eat at David's insistence. My face was pinched and I had deep frown lines. I felt my mother's eyes on me, and David's, too. Their gazes hurt. I didn't want their company and was too restless to be alone. I didn't go outside. I couldn't bear to see life going on, people smiling, oblivious to my suffering; mothers and fathers with children—families.

It was snowing the day of my pregnancy test. The usual noise outside my window was hushed.

I put on my high boots and a long coat. I was overcome with eagerness as I found a cab and went to Dr. Owins's office. There was an eerie stillness in the empty city streets and my heart was pulsating in my head.

The office was in a brownstone, down four steps. As I walked down, my boot caught on the hem of my coat. I tripped and slid down the icy stairs, landing heavily on my knees in front of the door. If I had been pregnant, I certainly wasn't now, I thought. I could barely walk; my legs hurt and my body felt clammy. I tried to collect myself before checking in for my pregnancy test.

"We'll call you at three o'clock," the nurse said after drawing blood. I gave her my number at Sambuca.

I knew I wasn't pregnant.

JENNIFER TOLD ME the first six months of her second pregnancy were the best part of her relationship with Stephen. He was attentive and willing to do anything to see her smile and acknowledge him. She had learned to have faith in him.

But Stephen was putting on a valiant front for his wife. At thirty-nine years of age and unemployed, he was facing a personal crisis. He got up each morning and dressed for job interviews. He told his wife that he was unable to find a place for himself with an adequate salary that would afford him self-esteem. Things changed when he refused to go back to the media business. Jennifer was horrified; worst of all, he looked to Stanley to help him find an opportunity in New York City. Jennifer told Stephen she would go anywhere with him but New York.

He ignored her pleas, went to New York, and invested in a new branch of Stanley's cousin's medical supply company.

Stephen's severance money was soon exhausted, what with a court order to continue child support, a mortgage on the house, a loan from Stanley, and overdue taxes. Jennifer was forced to put her house on the market.

While Stephen was in New York, she remained in Chicago until the house was sold. Hilary was her Lamaze coach. When Jennifer was in labor she called Stephen, who flew home in time to see Austin born. He was born vaginally, without C-section, as Kodie had been; Jen told me she willed it. "I wanted to feel what it was like to give birth rather than being laid out on an operating table with IV dripping into my strapped-down arms and having the baby taken from me. With the C-section I was so drugged on morphine I couldn't even hold Dakota right away."

A month later, Jennifer brought her two children to New York. She was devastated. She and Stephen were forced to live on her salary and inheritance. They took a small apartment in Queens; she hired a baby-sitter and went back to selling television time. Her salary was higher than Stephen's.

David and I tried to be with them, but I was working and Jen was working and commuting. There was no time. Now she says, "I was a hateful person and didn't want to be near anyone." My mother spoke to her, but felt Jennifer was pushing her away.

Jennifer's excuse was: "Liza, you have your mother, I don't have mine." It was not unlike the way she acted as a teenager. Over the years, Jen had been eager to share her joys, but during times of personal crisis, she would withdraw and push me away. It is an amazing contrast to how fervently she rises to the occasion when I am in need. She ignores her own advice to share problems with those who offer support. In this way, she pushed her husband out of her life.

Life in New York was unbearable for Jennifer. Stanley had remarried. I believe she felt he abandoned her. She secured a job in Chicago, bought a small town house for herself and her children, and moved back. Four months later, Stephen realized the medical supply business was a mistake. He, too, went back to Chicago and moved in with his father. This time he did get a high-paying job in the media business, which he knew well and where he could be productive.

In three months' time, when Stephen could contribute to family expenses, Jennifer let him move into the house with her. They were again a functioning family.

"What made you decide to go back with Stephen?" I asked, wanting to penetrate the barrier she had thrown up around herself.

"I don't want to break up my family. I never did. I had to find a way to gain back respect for Stephen. Liza, when he lost his job and cowered instead of fighting back and getting another position in the business where he was respected, qualified and insisted on moving to New York to start a business he knew nothing about, I couldn't look at him."

"Insisting on New York is where he made a mistake."

"He lost sight of everything. Stephen has been in one field all his life. He had no experience with medical supplies. How could he establish and operate a business he knew nothing about?"

"You told me before, he wanted what Stanley had—a business of his own, without being dependent on someone else for a job. I can understand that, after working so hard and being fired because of downsizing. That's scary for a man with a large family to support."

"Liza, I told Stephen I'd go anywhere in the world with him but not New York. Not where all I have are memories of Mommy. He didn't listen, and he didn't open his eyes to reality. It takes time to make a new business lucrative. Years. And he owed money to his ex-wife for child support. I was tired of taking care of everyone. I wanted to be done with that, and have someone care for me. I needed to be taken care of."

"Like your mother did," I said flatly.

"Yes. I'm not ashamed to say it. Stephen let me down. Therapy helped me be able to say it, and it helped me understand Stephen."

"You went together for a long time."

"That's how we learned to communicate. I had been cruel, making judgments without understanding, and he didn't listen to what I said, beyond my words. Neither of us made the effort to help the other. Now, with therapy, we have."

"You've done the right thing for yourself, and for Stephen and for Kodie and Austin. Maybe, with understanding, you'll put this problem behind you. You wouldn't want to raise two children alone."

"The way Mommy did? Never."

"Let me tell you—you were a vicious human being. Now your voice has changed; it has the commitment it used to have. You've never failed at what you set yourself to do."

"I couldn't get my mother well."

"Jen, you made her happy and gave her a grandchild. She knew Kodie."

"It will take time with Stephen. It isn't a job I can call finished, I know that. But now Stephen and I have a peaceful meeting ground."

Within four months, they were able to buy another house in Lake Forest, and were living again as a family—separate individuals, conscious of each other's weaknesses and strengths and united through all diversity.

When Austin was a year old, Greg's wife, Maxine, had a daughter—Sophia. Greg now had two children.

It was my turn.

I was not pregnant. When Dr. Holbrook called to confirm my belief, I felt a tremendous pain in the back of my head, as if I'd been hit without warning from behind. I thought I had prepared myself for a negative result. My mind, it seemed, was prepared, but once again, my body was not in sync with my head. I felt my insides cave in. The cycle at Fairfax had failed.

"Could it have been the fall down the few steps that caused me to lose the pregnancy?" I asked Dr. Holbrook. I didn't want to believe all that David and I had invested had been ruined by the slip of a foot.

"No," she said. "It was either poor cell division or your body rejecting the embryo. The immunological factor. Liza, you weren't pregnant."

We were still scheduled to begin an IVF cycle at Cornell in October, seven months from then. I wanted to believe there was still hope for us with IVF. Dr. Holbrook had said every attempt did not result in pregnancy; she also emphasized that IVF was still experimental. I didn't know what to do.

Chapter

16

A week had passed since the pregnancy test. My knees and back were stiff and ached from the fall, but I was barely conscious of it.

I had thrown myself into working. I was at the restaurant by 11:00 A.M. to receive deliveries and left after closing at midnight.

David also kept himself busy. From the office he went to the gym, and was never home before nine-thirty. He would order in dinner for himself. By the time I got home, he was often sleeping.

We had no communication, but we understood each other and knew it was best to leave the other to their own route of escape.

Patricia reminded us of the donor-sperm option. I could be inseminated without going through another IVF cycle, which I surely wanted to avoid. I could be treated privately by Dr. Owins, who had assisted me before we went to Fairfax—no IVF, no large hospital. I would be given Clomid, in pill form.

Clomid causes the pituitary gland to release hormones that stimulate the ovaries to produce more eggs. It is prescribed for women whose ovaries and glands are functioning normally but require a boost.

On Clomid, my menstrual cycle would not be shut down as it had been with Lupron. In conjunction with the Clomid, I would have to use heparin as a prophylactic, because Clomid, too, thickens the blood. Because David's immature sperm could only be injected into eggs retrieved from IVF, we would use donor sperm.

Neither of us was wholly convinced that donor sperm was an acceptable compromise. I felt very weird at the prospect of a stranger's sperm being put into my body . . . to have a baby that would be half of me and half of a faceless #2047 . . . too short but with a high IQ. David would have no genetic part in the child. Was that fair after all this?

We still were unsure whether we would tell everyone about the donor sperm or not. We could always say that we implanted frozen sperm from a previous cycle and no one would suspect. This way we could keep our options open and maintain some privacy.

Living a lie is not something David and I were comfortable with, but we did not know which way would be best for the child: believing he was the biological son of both his mommy and daddy or living with the knowledge that his biological father was a mystery.

We decided for now not to tell people about the donor sperm.

The psychology of adoption was simpler for me. David and I would be equal if we chose adoption.

David held to his original intent. "If it can't be my sperm, at least it will be my wife's egg."

So we agreed to a Clomid cycle.

Patricia Greene, our infertility counselor, like me, was a strong advocate of telling the truth. "It is better to avoid the possibility of the truth leaking out and breaking a trust. Love is trust and the foundation on which a family should be built."

Some women on Clomid experience hot flashes or cramps and breast tenderness. I had a constant headache. The Clomid, it was explained, fools the body into thinking blood estrogen levels are low, as in menopause, thus stimulating the same unpleasant effects.

I didn't suffer from the severe mood swings I had when I was on Lupron, but I didn't respond well to Clomid. I had only two eggs. I was artificially inseminated; #2047 and my eggs were united. I didn't know if I wanted it to work. Did I want a baby with a catalog number for a father? Would David and I tell the truth or not?

In two weeks, we were able to do a home pregnancy test. It was negative and I was strangely relieved. The doctors gave the reasons: inadequate eggs and poor cell division, or the immunological factor. The fault was not with the donor sperm. Number 2047 had successfully sired many offspring. The fault, then, could not be in David's sperm, since the results were the same even after that factor had been removed. The fault was mine.

Both Dr. Holbrook and Dr. Owins suggested we try again.

"Enough!" I said. No more tricks to my body or to me. I went back to work and found that if one is adamant enough, it is the mind that truly controls the body. I took myself out of the infertility picture. I put our October appointment for IVF at Cornell out of my mind and paid no attention to the looming date. Like Scarlett O'Hara, I'd think about it tomorrow.

Chapter

17

*O*n a hot Monday morning in August, I was in the city, hating being there, and hating the work that made it impossible for me to enjoy the ocean breezes. David had gone to work and I was sipping coffee, gazing out the window at the dense humidity and pollution.

For months, I had been bothered by stiffening joints and back pain. Even my fingers ached. I couldn't sit through an entire movie. David, tired of my complaining and my excuses that it would go away, insisted I see our family doctor. My appointment was for eleven A.M. I finished my coffee and got ready to jump into the shower.

The phone rang. I picked it up knowing it was Jennifer; she always called at this time to chat about the night before or plans for the day.

"Liza." Her tone was unusually enthusiastic. "I'm on my way to work, the traffic is awful, and I just figured out how you can have your baby."

"Jen, please, I'm trying to put it out of my mind for a while. I don't—"

"But, La," she burst in. "I have the solution. You and I can fix it. We can do it."

"Do what, Jen? I really don't want to think of IVF or infertility."
I was getting annoyed. "I'm going to be late for my doctor's appointment. Right now I just want to find out why I can hardly straighten up in the morning."

"Liza, I'll carry your baby!" She blurted it out as if it were the most natural thing in the world.

"Now I know you're nuts."

"Why can't the embryo—your egg, David's sperm—be transferred into my uterus? Your biological child!"

"It sounds sensible, but it's too crazy to even think about."

"Liza, pregnancy is easy for me. I'm at my most gorgeous. I like my stomach getting round with life and the admiring, knowing glances from passersby. I feel beautiful and I'm not afraid of giving birth. La . . . I'll carry your baby."

"Jen, I know we've had two failures at IVF. But it hasn't been determined that it's impossible for me to carry a baby. The doctors keep encouraging me to try again and we have that scheduled IVF cycle at Cornell coming up in two months. They've had more successes at live births than any clinic. I told you, my neighbor is about to have twins, after years of trying."

"Then why didn't you go there in the first place?"

"Because David's urologist referred us to Mount Sinai's clinic. But Jen . . . thank you, I know you say it out of love."

"Call me crazy, but you'll have a baby one way or the other. It might as well be the best possible way—your egg, David's sperm, and me as the oven. We can do it."

"Do you know what you're saying? Have you thought about . . . being pregnant with someone else's child?

"I just thought about it and it's a firm offer. My children are the reason for my existence. I want you to know the same reason for being. Think about it. Gotta go, I'm at the garage."

She disconnected and I found myself dumbly staring at the receiver in my hand. "Nonsense," I whispered, and hung up.

It was an innocent offer, spoken in pure love and ignorance of what carrying my child entailed. The term for Jen's solution, I found out later, is "gestational carrier." Jennifer offered to be the gestational carrier for me and David without either of us knowing the word or what was involved medically and emotionally. We were ignorant of what it would do to David and me to see our baby growing in Jen's body, and the self-imposed debt it would incur. Ignorant of how she would feel giving up the child she had carried and whispered to and felt kick and form inside her. And how her own children, Kodie and Austin, knowing the baby in their mother's womb was not their brother or sister, would react. And to think that she would give the baby away! What nightmares would arise for those children? Would their mother give them away, too? It was a thought spoken in ignorance of how her husband would feel about not being able to be intimate with his wife because she was carrying a child that wasn't his. What would happen to their marriage, which had almost been destroyed already and needed nurturing?

I told David. He looked at me quizzically as I related the conversation over spaghetti dinner at our kitchen table. "Naive, yes," he said resting his fork on his plate. "But not so crazy. Logically it could be done, and it *is* another option. I don't know if we would want to do it. It's a beautiful offer. I don't understand it myself. Jennifer and I are close but that's a lot of love talking. You and I are a couple, so are she and Stephen. A gestational-carrier situation would be between all of us. What has Stephen to gain? You girls jump into things too readily, both of you. The idea is exciting, but how exciting would it be for each of us to live with for nine months? Have you thought of the repercussions? What if it fails?"

David had been talking as if to himself, pondering step-by-step as he did in his business. "What's involved medically?" he continued. "Financially? And legally? Have you thought of the legality? She and Stephen depend on a dual income. She didn't work when she was pregnant with Kodie or Austin, and she's older. Liza, all this is premature. And what if she gets sick or miscarries? We're set to start the IVF at Cornell in about three weeks. Let's keep our heads on straight."

Chapter

18

*F*or Jennifer's thirty-fifth birthday, Mom and I sent Stephen money to help him treat Jen to a four-day stay at the Canyon Ranch Spa in Arizona. She wanted to be by herself to seek relief from the pain of her mother's death, which she still hadn't accepted. She wanted to step away from her role as wife and mother and rediscover Jennifer.

She had been away for three days and hadn't called, which alarmed me, but then I received a most remarkable letter.

Dear Liza,
I am writing you this letter because it is easier for me to express myself on paper.

Here in Arizona I can see the power of creation in the ageless mountains and the desert. It shows me that despite upheaval, nature is made to go on and so must I. I sought hypnosis as a tool to find my own recreation. La, you know I have always been a spiritual person and believe our greatest source of power and productivity comes from the mind. It frustrates me that I haven't been able to use that power to find peace since Mommy's illness and death.

Hypnosis always intrigued me, but it seemed like hocus-pocus. Not here. In the desert there is continuity: the colors spread, change, and recede as shadows hour after hour, and I now perceive hypnosis as a way to tone my whole being.

I went to the private session believing that if I could see Mommy again I would be able to close that chapter of her death and begin another and bring a happy wife to Stephen and a real mother to my children instead of the short-tempered, half-involved shrew that I feel myself to be.

Liza, I've been such an angry, miserable person. My existence has been superficial since my mother's death. Only you know that I put on fronts, but my mind and heart are out there floating and searching and absent from any interaction with my life.

Let me tell you about the hypnosis. I met the instructor in a darkened room and was told to lie back on the recliner. He sat behind me, out of sight. I surprised myself that I was able to relax and listen to his voice. You know me, I'm such a control fanatic. But his voice was soft and direct and it seemed like an anchor, I felt safe, and closed my eyes.

His voice led me through a labyrinth of hallways and doors. It was becoming monotonous. Then I saw Mommy. Liza, I saw her! And I heard her. She walked toward me carrying a bright light. Her face was so lovely, she was smiling, she looked happy. She handed me the light. I touched her beautiful hands. Her hands always meant so much: long, delicate fingers that could hold the world and give it to me. "Take the light, Jengi, carry it in your heart, know I live inside you." She said those words to me and then she moved away. I called after her, "Mommy." But, Liza, she moved farther but I still had the light and I didn't feel alone, or that she had been snatched away from me. Her going was gentle.

"I have you, Mommy, thank you. I love you," and then she was gone. But I smelled her perfume the way she promised. She really was there with me, Liza, I know I was with my mother. I want you to believe that. You are the closest one to me, different from Kodie and Austin and Stephen, you are my sister.

We are of the same origin and have shared the same times. You know me longer and better than anyone. Maybe better than I know myself. I think I know you better than you know yourself.

When I opened my eyes I wasn't in a daze. I was clearheaded, and felt a warmth in my heart, where there had been a stone. I couldn't wait to tell you. I almost called, but as I said, it was better to write.

Now I am going to take a walk and think what Mommy wants me to do with the light. My first thought and instinct is that she wants me to pass the light to you, La. I want to carry your baby. I say that with the deepest sincerity. We will do it together. You will cure my pain and I will cure yours. Then you and I can stand together and stop being the hateful brats we are.

I love you,
Jen

Had I been there that Sunday night I would have seen Stephen pick Jennifer up at O'Hare Airport. He had been leery of the mood he'd find her in, but her eyes were shining for the first time since Austin's birth. She kissed him warmly and embraced him, and Stephen was sure she had missed him. He held her at arm's length. "You look great. I'm glad you went if you come back to me happy and looking like this."

They got into the car and Stephen eased into the traffic moving out of the airport.

"I know you aren't a believer, Stephen," she said, trying unsuccessfully to contain herself, "but I saw Mommy under hypnosis." She watched his face sag. Quickly, so as not to discourage him, she took his hand, but revelation took precedence over his insecurity. "I honestly believe with my heart and mind that I have found a way to recover from her death, a way that will bring tranquillity and security to us as a family. Stephen . . ." She took a deep breath. "I'm going to have Liza and David's baby. It's meant to be. Liza doesn't know it yet, but I'm so sure of it." She opened the car win-

dow and shouted to the world. "I'm going to give Liza her baby."
She turned to her husband. "Will you take care of a wife who's
pregnant with someone else's baby, a woman who needs a lot of
attention? Will you be my partner?"

Jennifer had made up her mind and hoped Stephen would be
agreeable. There was no room for discussion. She regarded herself
as an independent person, and though she was functioning within a
marriage, she still had her own priorities.

She was relieved to see her husband laughing, and laughed with
him. It felt good, after so much misery—her mother's death and
their seven-month separation—to join in laughter.

For Stephen, it was thrilling just to see his wife so elated. He realized that she needed him to promise to be her partner. He wanted to
be needed, and for the sake of his family's harmony, he agreed to her
idea.

"I can't say I believe in signs, but if you do and you have at last
found relief, Jen, we'll look into it. I can't imagine not being a
daddy, not loving and having my children run to me. If I couldn't
have a child, I would exhaust every possible option. I would want
someone to do it for me." He touched her hand. "Jen, let's investigate everything about it and think of what it will mean to our
lives, to Austin and Kodie. She's old enough to understand an explanation. Liza isn't certain yet that she can't get pregnant. I'm your
life partner, but we have to realize there would be consequences.
We're a family. You and I have a responsibility first to our family.
There is more than having a baby involved."

Jennifer hadn't heard a word he said after he agreed to be her
partner; her mind was racing.

She felt like the old Jennifer, who got excited about things quickly
and acted on impulse. She was the wild Jennifer, dancing outra-
geously at the discos. She was the Jennifer who loved life and made
things happen instead of waiting for them to happen.

"What do I do with my body is my business," she told me later
when we had a chance to talk quietly and her initial exuberance had
given way to a more rational state of mind. "I wouldn't cheat on

my husband; that's a moral issue, I respect myself and him, I wouldn't do that. Having your baby, Liza, I am sure in my heart and soul, would make me a fit wife and mother and most important, a healthy human being. You said the idea of my being your gestational carrier is crazy. For your sake, I hope it doesn't come to that, but if you find out you can't carry a baby, I know you'll investigate it to the fullest."

"Jen, you are connecting this too much with your mother. This infertility problem, as it stands right now, is between David and me. I don't want to feel that I'm denying you the life preserver you need, but I can't encourage you. We are going to begin the IVF cycle at Cornell at the end of the month. I want it to be successful."

We hung up and I sensed I had disappointed her. She had wanted me to participate in her elation. Maybe it was similar to the times I let her down so sorely in high school and at college when she depended on me to introduce her to people and I didn't, but I didn't believe that wholly. Jennifer was a mature woman and knew herself. I believe she truly felt that giving me a baby would, in some way, even the score between the forces of life and death.

Chapter

19

*T*he fall foliage had reached its peak that final weekend of October 1996. I was tired. My joints ached, especially my knees. My family doctor had found no reason for these pains. I assumed my body was getting back at me for all the tricks I had played on it, even though I was told my discomfort was unrelated to IVF. I wasn't ready for the letter I received from the Cornell Infertility Clinic telling me to come in for my precycle consultation, consent form, pretesting, and schedules. The time on the wait list was over. My number had come up.

AT SIX O'CLOCK, Sunday afternoon, the Long Island Expressway westbound to New York City was living up to its reputation as the state's biggest parking lot. Traffic was at a standstill and I was in a black mood. David had put up with it all weekend, comforting me during my teary outbursts and stoically suffering my wicked tongue. We'd been in the car, sitting in silence, for almost two hours and weren't halfway to New York City. I was dreading the upcoming IVF cycle at Cornell. My appointment was in ten days. I still couldn't sit through a movie without having to get up and walk around the theater because of stiffness in my back. Looking ahead to a third IVF cycle with any hopefulness was impossible.

We were creeping toward Exit 49 in Huntington. "Turn here, David. I can't sit in the car any longer. Let's just go to Greg's and drive home later when this mess is over."

"How do you know he's home? We can't just drop over."

"He's my brother, for God's sakes. Of course we can go there. I know he's home, he's cooking dinner tonight. Turn! Turn here!"

David turned. I directed him past the malls in Oyster Bay and into Lloyd Harbor. He wound his way up Snake Hill Road beneath the high canopy of falling autumn leaves as I looked down the long driveways, trying to get a glimpse of the houses hidden behind stone walls and bushes. After fifteen minutes we pulled into Greg's driveway. It was almost dark, but I could still see Long Island Sound sparkling behind his white Colonial house.

Stuart ran out to meet us. "Aunt La!" I hugged him. A rugged seven-year-old, he looked like a little Greg. The same fathomless dark eyes and tousled black hair. No one could mistake the relationship between Greg, Stuart, and me. Stuart is warmhearted and sensitive like his father and has that same square smile that is so endearing.

Greg and Max came out on the porch with Sophia, now two years old, toddling behind. Sophia also looked like Greg, only she had Maxine's oval eyes.

Greg held a wooden spoon in one hand and a glass of red wine in the other. "I hope you guys are here for dinner. I'm making linguini with shrimp marinara sauce. There's plenty."

Max poured wine for me and David.

"I'll build a fire," David said, and stacked the logs in the fireplace behind the table in Greg's well-equipped work kitchen.

I was glad for the wine. Being with the kids cheered me up.

Greg held Sophia in his arms at the stove and let her stir the tomato sauce. Max was at the sink washing vegetables for salad, her blond hair held back in a ponytail, exposing her blue slanted eyes and full mouth. She had been working hard to lose the weight she'd gained from pregnancy. Her face had lost its puffiness and she was now proud of the way her body looked in tight jeans. My body was sore and would soon be even more sore and swollen in those same ugly elasticized skirts I had to wear, and after the whole torturous ordeal, I wouldn't have a little Sophia or Stuart in my house. Such were my thoughts.

"Aunt La. Come to my room and I'll show you my computer," Stuart said, pulling me by the hand.

"He has a computer?" I asked Greg.

"Yup."

"Stuart, you know how to work a computer? I'm amazed. Let's go!" I got up, took my wineglass, and followed him upstairs.

Stuart's room was a boy's paradise. He slept in a red racing-car-shaped fiberglass bed that had been Greg's. It still had the "Wetson's Racing Team" decal on the side. There were forts and trucks and shelves of matchbox cars and Lego constructions that he had built. The computer was on a desk with two red swivel chairs in front of it.

We sat down and Stuart lit up the screen with something called Math Blaster.

"You have to figure out the right equation to blow up that space creature," he explained, taking the mouse to demonstrate.

"I just learned to use the computer in my restaurant." I put the wineglass down on the desk out of the way.

"Aunt La. When you have your kid, you'll have to teach him the computer. Here." He gave me the mouse. "Choose from the multiple choices."

I picked the wrong equation and the monster advanced.

"When are you having your baby, Aunt La?"

"Stuart, how do you know about that?"

"My dad tells me. I know you're sad. But you should be happy."

He sounded so mature; Stuart was included in family conversations and his parents encouraged and listened to his opinions.

"You have people to help you, Aunt La." He jumped up and pointed to the screen. "Look! Another monster. Get that monster!"

I took the mouse and this time the monster was, as Stuart said, "history."

Greg came into the room. He had heard us talking. "Stuart, Mommy needs you downstairs."

Greg often took Stuart to work with him on weekends and let him help in the restaurant kitchens. He would peel carrots and fill ramakins with coleslaw, which made him feel important.

"Aunt La. You can play till I get back." He went downstairs.

Greg lay down on his old bed, crossed his feet, and put his hands behind his head. "Stuart's right, Liza. You're lucky to have the technology to help you. There are lots of women out there who don't have the money or live where they can't take advantage of the medical technology. A lot of women wish they were in your shoes."

I took a sip of wine. "I hate all those doctors. They don't care about me. They use women for their experiments. I hate their technology. I wish they didn't have it and that I didn't have to do this."

"You're just looking at it the wrong way. You're so fortunate to have these opportunities, and to be able to afford them. You have to change your outlook. Good things happen when you believe they will. The way your mind is now, you're defeated before you begin."

"And how do I change my mind?" I challenged, sipping the wine.

"Look at each day and think of three things to be positive about. It's a mental trick. If you ask your mind, 'What am I happy about?' you have tricked it into thinking of happiness and then you'll come up with things that make you happy. You like to be in control. Control your mind. If you tell yourself the technology and technicians are there to help you, then that's what they will do. And if you tell yourself that what you are doing you're doing with all your energy, heart, and soul, and therefore it must come out right, chances are it will. Even Stuart knows that."

My brother's words made me feel ashamed of myself. I had been indulging in self-pity again. "Thanks for the wake-up call," I said. "It was a much-needed one. I've forgotten who I am and what I'm capable of."

"Come on, pull me out of this bed before I fall asleep. Can you believe Max and I slept in this bed for over a year before we were married? Remember? Do you think Mommy knew?"

"Probably, but what could she do to stop you?"

We both laughed as I pulled him up by the arm. Superstitious as I am, I touched the bed hoping for the same luck it gave Greg and Max, then went down for pasta.

Delicious pasta . . . happy to be around my brother and his beautiful family . . . a wonderful husband, I thought. That's three good things today.

20

*A*fter the weekend, just a few days before my appointment at Cornell, I went to see a rheumatologist. The pains in my knees and elbows were impossible to ignore. My family doctor referred me to a Dr. Billings.

Before the examination, he asked me endless questions and punched my responses into a computer. I had never seen this before. It was annoying and impersonal. He asked me what I did. Did I work? What exercises and sports do I do? He asked about my family history and my physical history. I told him about the mini-stroke. He asked me if I had children and I told him about the failed IVF cycles and that I had been on the blood thinner heparin during these treatments.

At these last words, his fingers stopped on the keyboard. He looked at me with concern. "Do you know you are at great risk doing IVF with your blood condition? If you get pregnant, you would be putting yourself in serious danger of another stroke, or worse. No one told you?"

"I was told I'm a high risk, but they said the blood thinner would act as a prophylactic and prevent the hazards of blood thickening."

"I don't agree." He stood up angry. "Considering your anticardiolipin antibody syndrome, you shouldn't be trying to get pregnant with IVF or even normally. It would be life threatening."

He examined me and said my joint pain was caused by calcium deposits. As I left the office, Dr. Billings put his arm over my shoulder.

"Liza, this is off the record, but if you were my daughter I wouldn't allow you to be pregnant."

He scared me. I wanted another opinion. I felt that such a strong statement about my blood condition should come from a hematologist, a blood specialist, not a rheumatologist.

Considering the nature of the IVF cycle at Cornell, I asked to be referred to a hematologist on their staff so the blood and the infertility team could confer together and I wouldn't have to act as a "general contractor." Coincidentally, the hematologist told me that my particular condition was something that a rheumatologist would understand. He even referred me to another rheumatologist at Cornell.

After much testing and trying to get all of the doctors to compare notes Dr. Billings's opinion was confirmed; it could be quite dangerous for me to carry a baby. It was concluded that my anticardiolipin antibody level, the medical term for the blood-clotting condition, had prompted the transient ischemic attack I had in 1992. The doctors felt that the anticardiolipin antibodies combined with high estrogen levels and childbirth could cause a severe stroke.

I was outraged. How could they discover this now?

I could have died? How could they say this to me two years later? After all we'd been through? How could I trust another doctor? They were all idiots. David had had two surgeries. For what? His sperm could fertilize an egg. Why hadn't any one of the doctors looked at our full health picture? I had told them of my blood-clotting condition and the mini-stroke, and they had minimized it, focusing only on getting us pregnant. I was furious. And now what? What do David and I do?

We met with Patricia Greene and she brought up the idea of a gestational carrier. "Embryos of Liza's eggs and David's sperm would be transferred into another woman's uterus who would carry and give birth to the child. David, you and Liza would be the biological parents." We told her of Jennifer's offer. It seemed the dream could become a reality, a blessing in this time of hopelessness. Jennifer could be our gestational carrier. Jennifer, who'd offered to make this sacrifice without even knowing if such a procedure was feasible, without ever hearing the medical name for it—Jennifer could carry our embryo, and give birth to a child that would be created with David's sperm and my egg, our complete biological child.

Patricia answered many of the questions David had initially asked me. The gestational carrier would be put on hormonal therapy to get our menstrual cycles to coincide. She would not be given hormones to stimulate the ovaries to produce multiple eggs, but to suppress her ovaries so they would not produce her own eggs, and make her uterus receptive to the embryos. In other words, her body would function as if it were pregnant. There would be many preliminary tests, even a test cycle and biopsy of the endometrial lining of the uterus to ensure that she could support the embryo. And we would have to research the legalities in Illinois and New York.

Yes, this was a blessing, but it opened the door to many obstacles. It involved other people, as David had pointed out to me when I had first told him. There was much for David and me to consider before we spoke to Jennifer. If using a gestational carrier was possible perhaps we would seek a stranger, thereby avoiding personal feelings and long-term family involvement. Perhaps this would minimize the emotional complexities and pitfalls.

But then again, to have Jennifer carry our baby as a gift of love might, after all, be the most beautiful blessing of all.

Early Monday morning the phone rang. It would be Jennifer with her weekend report.

I had to interrupt her. "Jen, I have a doctor on the other line. I'll call you back at work . . . sorry." I hung up and listened to the obstetrician confirm the inauspicious results of my blood test; pregnancy could potentially cause a stroke.

Before the shock of that telephone call set in, I urgently called Jennifer at her office. Her assistant answered on the first ring.

"Ellen, is Jennifer busy? I've got to speak to her."

"She's away from her desk. Hold on, I'll get her for you."

In a moment Jennifer was on the line. "What'd the doctor say?"

With complete panic in my voice, I blurted out, "I shouldn't be pregnant because of my blood condition. I could have a stroke . . . or die."

"Liza, I was serious about the offer I made." She spoke without hesitation. "Let me carry your baby. Let's find out more about it."

"It's so complicated, Jen. I know about it; I spoke to Patricia, our infertility counselor. She told me the gestational carrier has to go through a lot of testing, and hormone therapy—all those awful injections. It's a major commitment."

"I know it's not simple. I want to do it. Set up an appointment. I'll come to New York and we'll meet with the doctor together."

"Jennifer, why would you do this for us?" I said with love, fear, and confusion.

She thought awhile, not because her answer was unclear, but to choose the words that would best express her feelings. "My mother's death and your mother's accident were all beyond our control. Since that time, each of us has been suffering. This is fixable. This is something we can accomplish together. When I give you the baby, I'll be left knowing I *gave* life. Not that it was taken from me. I'll experience love again and trust it. Now I fear it. Giving you the baby will give me joy. If I can give you the feeling of purpose and the incredible love my children have given me, I will make a difference in your life, and by letting me do this . . . that will make difference in my life."

I was moved by her words, but still I argued. "Jen, it's not just being pregnant. It's the whole in vitro cycle, plus psychological testing. There would even be a trial in vitro cycle to determine if you could carry the embryos. You saw what those drugs did to me. You would have to take all those drugs, all those shots and sonograms and blood tests—the endless visits to the doctor . . . besides, you're working. How could you do it?"

"We'll find a way."

"They have to make your body receptive and trick it into reacting as if it were pregnant. Jen, these drugs have side effects. Aside from making you feel as if the end of the world is upon us, and getting fat and uncomfortable, there could be kidney damage or other long-term effects. No one knows for sure; this technology is new. It's not just being pregnant; it takes over who you are and may cause tremendous stress in your family. You need to consider all this."

"La, I know I can do it, I know my two kids depend on me; this isn't a frivolous decision. I can do it. I'm not afraid. I see it as a finished thing. I see you with your baby."

"Jen, please, you don't have to do this. You're too brave and I'm afraid for you."

"Don't be. My mother wants me to give you the light. She wouldn't let harm come to me. Right now I need to take this aggressive step to survive."

"Are you aware of the magnitude of what you're saying?"

"I'm thinking of the outcome. Send me the information, but, Lollipop . . . this is meant to be."

After we hung up I was hysterically crying. I was overcome by the mysteries of love and the many unforeseen ways it can exert its power.

Jennifer saw carrying David's and my baby as an act of love, and David and I would be the beneficiaries of that love. I wanted to believe that a baby born out of so much love could only be a miracle.

Jennifer believed she has the power. My infertility created a challenge for her and she was rising to meet it. It answered a need in her nature to affirm life in general and her own committment to the forces of life. My dilemma could be the solution to her misery.

I called my mother immediately and told her about the proposal, saying "This opens up areas we can't even comprehend yet." She had been against drugs and IVF from the start, and had, for months, thought we would eventually opt for adoption.

"Liza, I want to share your happiness. There's nothing I wish for you more than to have your own baby—yours and David's. It's a good scientific plan, but there is no science to the multitude of emotions."

She called Jennifer at work and discussed it with her.

Jennifer said to me later, "I never heard your mother sound so strict. She told me I had to convince her that I was competent mentally and emotionally and would not endanger my health or my marriage. I gave her my word. She accepted it. I believe she wants this for us, she wants us to be careful, just as my mother does. We're not being foolhardy."

"Jen, did you tell Jack? You owe it to your brother to tell him and hear what he has to say."

"I tried to reach him and left messages on his answering machine. It's hard to track Jack down. He'll call me. He's probably out of town."

The next day I received a special-delivery letter:

Dear La,

Since I got home from Canyon Ranch, things have been moving so fast. Either you are busy at work or with doctors, etc. And me? I'm busy with my family and work.

I want to take time out to tell you, so you have no doubt, how committed I am to being your gestational carrier. It isn't for heroics or gratitude or because I think you are needy. It is because I think it is the right thing for me and for you and the baby you will have.

Aunt Suzy is trying to protect me. I know she is in a difficult position trying both to protect me and accomplish the most for you. It is a difficult role, for she is putting herself in Mommy's position. What would my mother say? All three of us know she would be the most enthusiastic. She is the reason for all these coincidences coming together at a time that is right in our lives. She orchestrated all these conditions so I would carry your baby, Liza. What better way for all of us to carry on? Could there be a stronger bond? It really doesn't matter to me what anyone else thinks but you. I want you to believe, as I do, and know the love flowing between us will bring success.

Love,
Jen

David and I read the letter over and over again. There was no ambiguity about Jennifer's motives, no doubt about the sincerity of her wish to carry our baby. For us it was the answer to a prayer, and in our hearts we wanted to rush into agreeing, but we still had reservations. I wrote a letter to Jennifer, trying to explain:

Dear Jen,

Your letter made me cry. I am trying to find words to express my feelings. I am searching deep in my heart and still, there are no words. I am frightened. I wish I was with you to hold you and have you hold me. It is a long untraveled road, and it is dark—we don't know what's out there. That's what frightens me, the unknown. But we have Aunt Laurie's light to follow.

I want so much to say, "Let's just do it." But I don't want anything to happen to you physically or emotionally. I don't want anything to happen to us. Oh, Jen, I want so desperately to say yes. We would be pioneers in a venture that connects people closer than blood.

Jen, now we must be rational. I know how positive you are, but you must consider the possibility of failure. No one guarantees any pregnancy will be healthy and carried to term. No one knows if the fetus will be healthy. What would happen if you miscarry or have to abort the child? I'm very concerned, Jen, about you. Would you feel you had lost another life? I know the very thought is painful, but we have to acknowledge it. A failure like that, out of your control, could be traumatic. Jen, that loss for you would be greater than the loss of an unborn child to me. There are no guarantees. Maybe it's best to avoid the possibility. If we succeed, would the gain be greater than the loss if we fail?

Because of the chance of failure, I have reservations. However, because you and I follow our hearts and because we love your mother's light, we will pursue this, Jen, all of us, cautiously, being fully informed and knowing medically what we are doing and what to expect. And emotionally, promising always to be truthful, and for you to know you can always change your mind.

I've called Cornell, at New York Hospital, and made our appointment with the head of the infertility clinic, Dr. Scot Gorin. The appointment is November 20, when you and Stephen and David and I will begin our in-depth education.

Until then, Jen . . . I, too, carry the light in my heart. It is life.

Love,
Liza

P.S. I am sending you some written material I received from the Cornell Clinic.

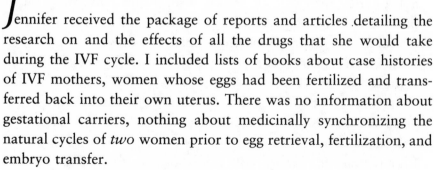

*J*ennifer received the package of reports and articles detailing the research on and the effects of all the drugs that she would take during the IVF cycle. I included lists of books about case histories of IVF mothers, women whose eggs had been fertilized and transferred back into their own uterus. There was no information about gestational carriers, nothing about medicinally synchronizing the natural cycles of *two* women prior to egg retrieval, fertilization, and embryo transfer.

We would be pioneers.

Jennifer studied the information and told me and Stephen, "Nothing bad is going to happen to us. Mommy is watching us. We'll be fine."

Each morning, as Stephen and Jennifer drove to work in downtown Chicago, they discussed the pros and cons of this mission. It would be something they would do as a family, in partnership with me and David. We would all sign a contract.

Jennifer touched her husband's knee. "My part would be to take extra precaution to safeguard the health of myself and the baby. Before, Stephen, when we were pregnant, we had unprotected sex. Now I'd insist you wear a condom. And Stephen . . ." She was teas-

ing him. "No extramarital partners allowed for either of us." She
laughed. "I say it as a joke, but you and I haven't been back together
for very long. It's a law that you and I take an AIDS test before I
begin IVF. We have to abide by a promise to prevent any chance of
contamination to ourselves and the fetus."

"Jennifer. With or without the belly, you're my only girl."

I received another letter from Jennifer. As often as we spoke on the
phone, she could express herself more candidly in letters.

Dear Liza,
Stephen and I went together to see my OB/GYN, Dr. Isola. She
delivered Kodie and Austin. She told me that though I had two
healthy pregnancies, each pregnancy is different. She said that
because I am older now, it might be more difficult to conceive
either naturally or with assistance. It seems thirty-five is not the
peak of childbearing years. I already knew this. I am not deterred. She couldn't tell me much about the drugs and said we
must get that info from the infertility clinic. I am looking forward to November 20.

We also went to see Arlene Kessler, my shrink. After four
years she has given me the confidence to look inward and be
able to be honest with myself, and I do rely on her guidance.
I know you are so very protective about your inner life, but I
was comfortable baring my soul with Stephen there. We've always been honest with each other since we got back together
and that's what kept us together. Arlene asked me why I am
doing this. There, with Arlene, I was able to say it clearly. I
told her, and Stephen, and I am writing this letter to tell you.
It is simple—a life has been taken from me and I want to create
one. I want to bring joy where there is suffering. I believe I can
do it, and when I have, I'll be able to move ahead. I told Stephen that once I accepted my mother's death by accomplishing
this, I will be free to be the wife he deserves and we will be a
family with happiness at its core instead of desolating grief.

It is my belief, Liza. I don't ask anyone's approval, but I do ask my husband to respect my faith in myself. I ask Arlene, who has taught me that strength and solace can only come from within, to support me. And I am pleased to say, they both comply with my requests.

Liza, I'll carry your baby. I will be well and give birth to a healthy child and Stephen will be my partner. We will be unified in a common goal, without judgment or guilt, and this goal will eradicate the doubt and accusations that separated us. It is the right thing for everyone.

Be assured, Liza, I am not approaching this lightly. We are going to have a healthy baby.

Love,

Jen

The letter was written by a woman whose eyes were open wide and who had looked at herself without comforting illusions. It was mature, straightforward, and honest. Jennifer had convinced me that she was acting intelligently and I felt confidence in her belief that she could suceed as our gestational carrier. As each of us weighed the pros and cons, it seemed to be the right decision.

*B*efore the fertility clinic at Cornell would even begin preliminary testing for the gestational-carrier cycle and transfer, we had to prove that pregnancy was not a viable option for me. As it happened, no fewer than four blood specialists could do this. However, Patricia informed us, psychological evaluation was also a requirement—not just for me but for David, Jen, and Stephen as well. There were also legal issues to consider.

Illinois law states that the woman who gives birth to a child is the legal mother, and her husband the legal father, unless she claims otherwise, and her claim can be proved genetically. Because of this, David and I would have to adopt the baby, a procedure that required the intervention of lawyers in Illinois as well as New York. We had moved into a new realm of the reproductive frontier.

Once again I found myself speaking to the serious, efficient women in doctors' offices who handle appointments. "This is Liza Freilicher, I'd like to speak with Dr. Scot Gorin." Patricia had referred me to him because he was the head of the department that dealt with gestational carriers. When I said the name out loud, I realized that I'd heard it before. Scot Gorin? I'd graduated from high school with a Scot Gorin. He had dated Jennifer. He was a cute guy on the varsity basketball team. When he got on the line, I couldn't resist asking where he was from.

"Woodmere, why?" the doctor asked.

"Do you know Liza Wetanson?"

"Sure. I went to school with her."

"I'm Liza!"

"Oh, my goodness. This is crazy! Liza, you're my patient?"

"And you'll never believe who my gestational carrier is. It's Jennifer—my cousin, Jennifer Luber."

"Jennifer? I can't believe it. I'll be so glad to see you."

We hung up. I was blushing and panicked. The following day, at nine A.M., I'd face Dr. Scot Gorin. Scot, who ordered strawberry-ice-cream sodas at the diner, who hid in my bathtub when the police came looking for the kids who'd thrown raw eggs at passing cars on Halloween. How could I let him give me a pelvic exam?

But having Scot as my new doctor was a good omen.

It was November 5, 1997. I will always remember the date as the day my life turned around and I began to have faith that I would be a mother. It was the day of my first appointment at the Cornell Infertility Clinic at New York Hospital.

I was relieved to find that Scot grasped the awkwardness of our predicament immediately. We laughed at the outlandish coincidence. He explained the entire process of gestational carrying to me.

Having Scot manage our cycle seemed like fate. He knew both Jennifer and me, he was part of our history, and today for the first time I felt I was being treated like a person, not just an infertility patient.

I remembered my talk with Greg up in Stuart's bedroom. I pictured my brother lying on that race-car bed telling me to think of three positive things. Three things, I commanded myself now. Jennifer's offer, Scot, and my ability to make things happen. I was already feeling more positive.

A technician took my blood and a radiologist did the hysterosalpingogram. The doctor was gentle; it hurt but not as much as I anticipated, probably because I was feeling more hopeful.

I hoped Jennifer would have an easy time. I wished she didn't have to go through the trial cycle, but she was not complaining about it. The more she learned, the more enthusiastic she became. I kept telling her: if anything becomes too intense, too scary or difficult, speak up and tell me. I did not want her to feel as if she had gotten our hopes up and then would let us down. Just the fact that she had offered to give us this opportunity was an amazing gift. I knew that Jen and I would carry on the tradition of our mothers for our generation of offspring.

It was ironic to me: when David and I began seeing infertility doctors, my reproductive system was given a clean bill of health. It was David's sperm that was the problem. Suddenly it was my blood condition that was preventing me from becoming pregnant. I was confused about not being the birth mother of our child. During the IVF cycles and after the transfers, I dreamed of being pregnant. Now, though, with Jennifer being gestational carrier, David and I were equal again: my egg, his sperm.

I couldn't imagine how I'd feel seeing Jennifer pregnant, knowing it was my baby in her. I couldn't comprehend this miracle. They would be so far away—Jennifer and our baby in Chicago, David's and my baby growing inside my cousin. Could I say that I myself was having a baby? I could. I was, after all, the mother. I would play a large role in the birth of our child; intuitively, I would feel joy at every movement and suffer every one of Jen's discomforts, and send a tape of my voice for Jen to play so the baby would know it and be comforted inside the womb. And I would find a way to show Jennifer how much David and I loved her and appreciated what she was doing for us. Jennifer and I would be in sync, just as our cycles had been.

With my egg and David's sperm, an embryo inside of her, we were all three linked as one, with one goal—the birth of a healthy baby.

Chapter
23

I got out of bed on the morning of November 20 with the nervousness and excitement that come from not having slept the night before. Jen was going to meet me at the Cornell Infertility Clinic for our appointment with Scot. Ordinarily, I would have chosen to wear all black—my city wardrobe—but for this occasion I thought my gray pantsuit would make a positive statement. I felt as if I were moving in a rarefied atmosphere. I had been chosen to play a major role in a true-life historic drama.

David and I waited for Jennifer and Stephen outside the main entrance to New York Hospital. I stood beside the stone pillar watching each taxi and car discharge its passengers. I could tell who was a patient, who a visitor or employee. It was the set of the eyes and mouth. When Jennifer stepped out of the cab, I felt a surge of adrenaline. My heartbeat thundered in my ears. I ran to her. No words were needed, only contact. When we separated, each of us wiped her eyes and laughed, not at the silliness of our emotions but at the relief of being together and finally getting started. Then David and I, Jen and Stephen walked into the hospital.

The two of them were outstanding. In my eyes, they exuded a heroic radiance, and I felt that all who beheld them could sense that these two were embarking on a lofty mission. Stephen wore gray trousers and a black jacket. Jennifer was in a tailored charcoal pin-striped pantsuit with a black crepe tank top. Hanging from her neck, on a long chain, was an oval antique gold locket. Aunt Laurie, I remembered, wore that locket all the time. My mother had given it to her when Jennifer was born. Inside were photos of Jen and Jack. Now the locket carried pictures of Dakota and Austin. Jennifer touched the necklace. "Lollipop, you'll wear this with a picture of your baby inside."

Three positive things, I repeated to myself again. Jennifer, David, and me. I was convinced we would have this baby.

Before going into Dr. Scot Gorin's office, Jennifer pulled me aside. She whispered so Stephen wouldn't hear. "La, do you think Scot will examine me? I know he didn't examine you, but we're in a different position. Maybe he'll have to do the exam on me himself. Oh my gosh, I haven't seen him in twenty years and now I'll just be another uterus to him. I'm not changing my clothes and going in there with my feet in those stirrups before he sees me dressed. I mean that."

I didn't blame her. Lying on your back in clinical garb with your knees apart is no way to be confronted with an old high-school boyfriend, one who didn't get to "second base" with you.

We went into Scot's office, just Jen and I. Scot came in before we were seated. "You look wonderful," he said with due admiration.

Jennifer blushed. "You haven't changed."

We reminisced for a bit.

I couldn't wait to show Jen and Scot the old photos I'd managed to dig up after I spoke to him. There was one in particular of Scot with three of the cutest, most popular boys in our class; they were in the playground wearing some girls' coats they had stolen from under a tree. Scot was wearing my long, red-and-black plaid coat with the peaked hood.

We all laughed. Jen threatened to show the photograph to the entire world if Scot didn't get us pregnant.

It was nice to know that Scot was our friend and that he could be this without compromising his objectivity as a doctor.

He sat behind his desk, Dr. Scot Gorin. He told us what proce-

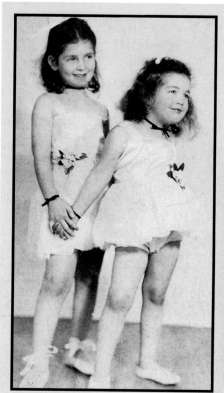

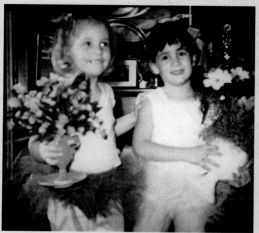

Suzanne and Laurie at a
ballet recital, 1942

Jennifer and Liza putting on a show
for family in Liza's den, 1966

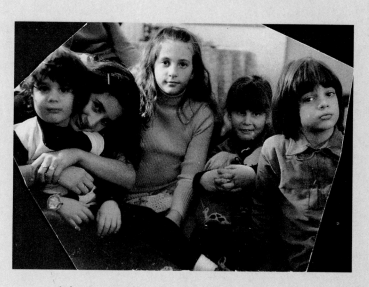

(left to right) Greg, Liza, Jennifer, Erica, and Jack
at their grandmother's house, 1971

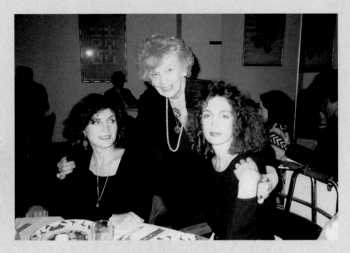

Suzanne, Grandma Reese, and Laurie at
Liza's birthday party, 1989

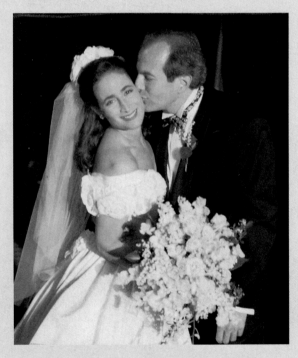

Liza and David's wedding photo, 1993

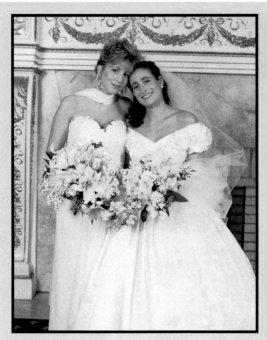

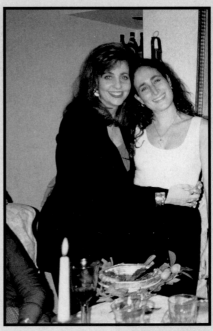

Jennifer as maid of honor at Liza
and David's wedding, 1993

Thanksgiving, 1996, the night
Jennifer and Liza and their husbands
decided that Jennifer would be
the gestational carrier

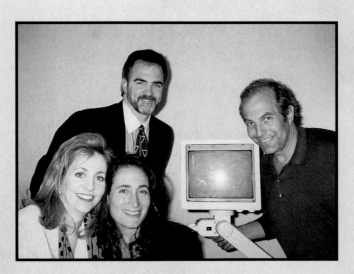

Jennifer, Stephen, Liza, and David at the amniocentesis,
June 1997; Luc can be seen on the monitor.

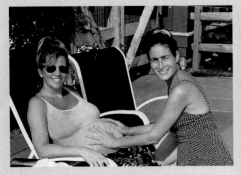

Liza with a very pregnant Jennifer,
August 1997

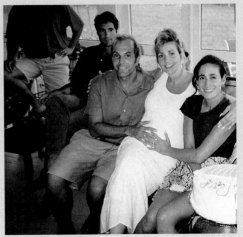

David, Jennifer, and Liza, at the
baby shower, August 1997

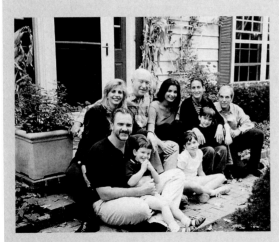

Jennifer's family in front of
Jennifer and Stephen's house
in Illinois, October 1997:
(left to right) Stephen, Jennifer,
his father, Ralph, her best friend,
Hilary, Liza and David, with
the children, Austin, Dakota,
and Michael

Liza, Jennifer, Stephen, and
David leaving for the hospital
at five in the morning, on Luc's
birthday, October 16, 1997

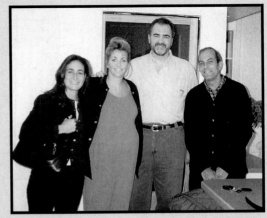

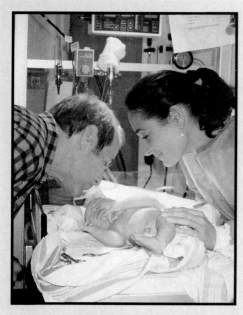

The proud parents inspecting
their beautiful baby,
October 16, 1997

Liza, Jennifer, and David
with Luc, October 16, 1997

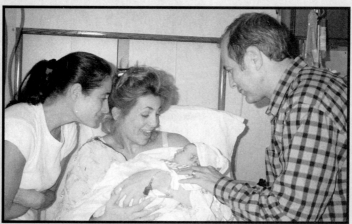

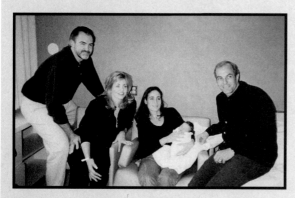

Stephen, Jennifer, Liza, Luc, and
David preparing to leave the
hospital, October 16, 1997

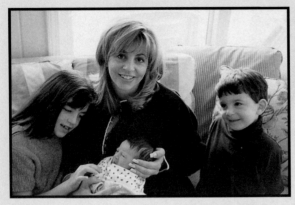

Jennifer with Dakota and Austin enjoying their newborn cousin before he goes home to New York, October 17, 1997

Liza and David carrying Luc over the threshold of his new bedroom, October 17, 1997

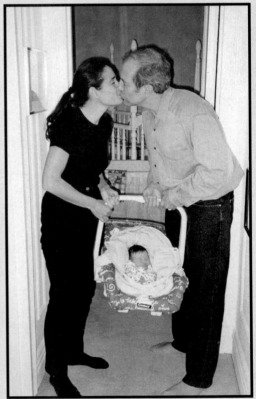

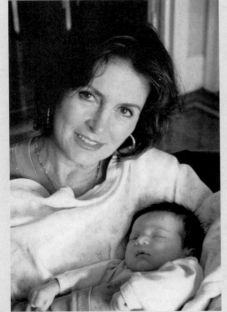

Suzanne with her newborn grandson, October 18, 1997

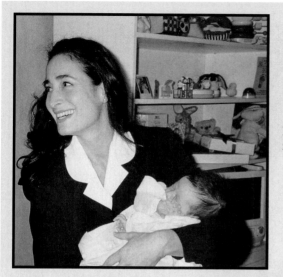

Liza and Luc in preparation
for his bris, October 26, 1997

A three–generational outing
in Central Park, October 30, 1997

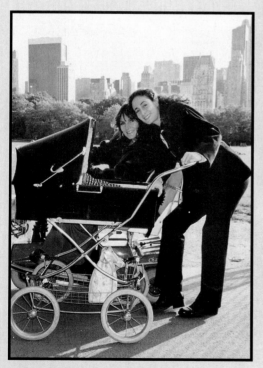

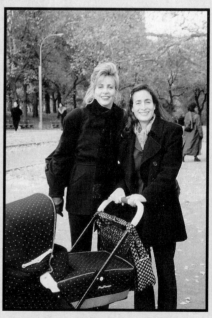

Jennifer and Liza
taking Luc for a stroll,
November 1997

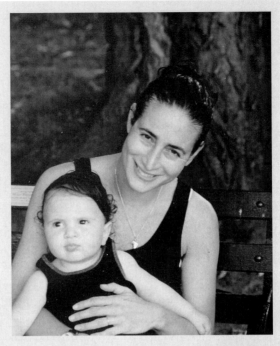

Liza and Luc, April 1998 *(Photo credit: Bob Woods)*

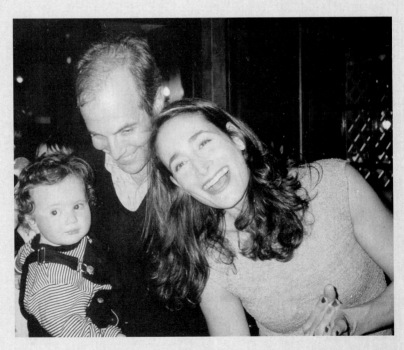

Luc's first birthday, October 16, 1998

dures and medicines were involved. I would have ovarian stimula-
tion to increase the number of eggs to be retrieved and thereby
increasing the chances of fertilization. Jennifer, the gestational carrier, would take various medicines during the cycle to prepare the
lining of her uterus to accept the embryos once they were transferred. Since the gestational carrier and genetic mother are not on
the same cycle, Lupron would be administered starting on day
twenty-one of the prior cycle. Once the cycles were stopped, the
hormones estrogen and progesterone would be given to the gestational carrier to prepare her uterus to receive the embryos. Estrogen
would be given as a skin patch, progesterone by daily injection for
twelve weeks of pregnancy—if pregnancy occured.

"First, a preparatory cycle must be performed to determine how
your body will react," Dr. Gorin explained. "In this cycle, we will
give you the same medications you will be receiving during the cycle
for the embryo transfer. Dosages have to be individualized. We will
check blood tests and possibly take a biopsy of your uterine lining,
an endometrial biopsy, to see if the uterus is properly prepared to
accept the fertilized eggs. The eggs will be retrieved and, in your
case, fertilized by ICSI. It takes a steady hand and a powerful mi-
croscope. Our team has both of these." He smiled and looked like
the old Scot again, warm and encouraging.

He continued. "As soon as we know how many eggs become
fertilized, we will let you know; it takes two days. Three days after
fertilization, a maximum of three embryos will be transferred to
reduce the risk of multiple births. Jennifer, you will rest here in the
hospital for half an hour and then go home and take it very easy.
Blood will be drawn eleven days following transfer to determine
your estrogen and progesterone dosages. If the test is positive, you
will continue the medicine and have biweekly blood tests and occasional ultrasounds to document the growth of the pregnancy. After twelve weeks, you will be referred to your obstetrician for
follow-up. Jennifer, because you live in Chicago, we will arrange for
your OB/GYN to take the blood tests, sonograms, and the endometrial biopsy and send us the reports."

I knew the procedure and had explained it all to Jennifer, but hearing it from a doctor's mouth made it sound so much more real and definitive. And then, too, I was so emotional about IVF because of my own experiences with it that I had not adequately conveyed the genuine rigors of the procedure.

"In addition," Scot went on, "there are risks to you, Jennifer. You and Liza and your husband must take HIV and hepatitis tests because these diseases are transmissible to the embryo."

"Whew," Jennifer said, "is that all? When this is over you'll have a positive statistic for your records."

Without the least embarrassment, Scot told Jennifer that he would do her pelvic exam because it was into her uterus that the transfer would be made and he had to know the configuration of her cervix and uterus.

Jennifer's expression remained set as she listened. Not for a moment did she reveal the awkwardness she had to have been feeling. Scot told her that after the exam she would go to the radiologist for a hysterosalpingogram. I wanted to go with her, but Scot said no, I was to wait here in the office.

Before following Scot out of the office, Jennifer turned to me and handed me a note. "Read this while you're waiting."

Then she walked beside Scot down the hall toward the examining room. I heard him introduce her to his nurse. The three of them laughed, seemingly at ease. Jen giggled at some joke of Scot's I wasn't able to hear.

I settled back in the chair facing Scot's desk in the empty office. I looked about at his many diplomas, and turned the standing picture frame on his desk around to see the photo of a fresh-faced young woman with loose long brown hair. In her arms was a young boy, and beside them a little blond girl, about Stuart's age, offering a bouquet to her baby brother. *For Daddy, we love you,* was written in childish penmanship across the bottom.

I opened Jennifer's note:

Dear La,
Here I am writing to you again; this time I'm in the plane and
I will soon be hugging you. La, we're moving forward together
to create a dream. In my dream, I see you and David and me

with the most treasured miracle of all—your child. It is strange; at this moment it is a dream, but when we meet and touch and the current flows between us, it will be real. Scot will have it documented. Today we start the creation. It seems so . . . gossamer but it isn't. It's tough, down-to-earth, today reality, and I can't wait.

Jen

Moved, I read the note over and over. Jen came back into the room. I wiped my eyes and breathed heavily.

"That's it. Done—the worst is over," she said, after the hysterosalpingogram.

After still more blood tests and exams, we waited to have a consultation with Scot. He answered questions about drugs, the anticipated effects, and explained that this trial cycle of Jennifer's would give a good preview of how her uterus would respond during the actual cycle. Because the gestational-carrier program at the infertility clinic at Cornell Medical Center was new, they had only three cases. Two were now pregnant and one was waiting to take her pregnancy test. Jennifer and I would be the fourth.

At three o'clock that same afternoon, we went for the psychological evaluation and tests. The dry turkey sandwich we'd shared in the cafeteria, however vile tasting, at least served to energize us.

"This is a joke," Jen said as we got off the elevator and looked for the psychologist's office. "Anyone can see we're all for it, one hundred percent. We're not holding anything back and we trust each other."

"Maybe the psychologist will bring up issues we haven't considered. It's another chance to make sure before we begin. I'm not against it. It will just reenforce our certainty."

"Look at David and Stephen," Jen said, turning around to look at our husbands following us. "They think we're crazy. Neither of them ever expected the four of us would be a team."

"It's like we are all four married." I laughed. "But they don't think we're crazy. They think we're strong."

•   •   •

David and I stayed in the waiting room outside the office while Jen and Stephen met with Joan Petit, the psychologist assigned to our case. We had our psychological evaluation weeks before. Now it was Jen and Stephen's turn.

After about an hour Joan asked us in to have a group meeting. Jen and Stephen were seated on the green tweed sofa. Jen gave me a glance that meant, "This is a ridiculous waste of time."

Joan Petit was a frizzy-haired matron who was wearing a burgundy jacket buttoned to her throat; it camouflaged whatever bosom she might have had. She seemed bitter and unfeminine looking, I thought. It was her job to determine whether we were all four in agreement, if we had the stamina and emotional balance to complete our undertaking, and if we could deal with any harmful repercussions that might arise after birth. I wondered if she was at all aware that love and fortitude as ours did exist.

We all hoped the interview would be useful and insightful. However, the questions were tedious and all seemed to concern physical ability or family history rather than emotional fitness. How many siblings do you have? Ages? Parents? Married? Divorced? Remarried? Education? Pregnancies? Deaths? Ethnic backgrounds? Heart disease? Cancer? Diabetes? Obesity? Drugs?

Nothing insightful was brought to light. It was, in all our opinions, a waste of time. Jennifer said she took particular offense at the woman.

"She never asked if Stephen and I had experienced marital problems. She concentrated on our siblings and relationships with our parents. Liza, she didn't even ask how we felt about our agreement; she never asked how you felt about not being pregnant or why I wanted to do this. Where is that woman's head? She's jealous. I think she's out to get us. I could tell by her eyes when she checked us all out. That witch could stand in our way and prevent us from realizing our dream."

Stephen reassured us that the psychologist was looking out for our well-being. "Jennifer," he said, "you would not have been given the hysterosalpingogram if they thought you wouldn't be approved. The psychological test was merely a formality."

"Well, that woman isn't competent to understand any of our feelings. She knows nothing. She knows nothing about Mommy. Look how long Arlene and I worked together. She knows. She's the one to judge. It infuriates me." Jennifer took a deep breath. "I sound paranoid, don't I? I'm overreacting. I'm tired."

Jennifer and I then had to take another psychological test, the Minnesota Multiphasic Personality Inventory. Only after the evaluation of the test and an okay from the psychological examiner could the gestational-carrier cycle begin. That was the law. Scot had told us about it during our consultation. It was annoying.

David went down to the lab for some blood tests and Stephen grabbed the *Times* while Dr. Petit handed Jen and me a huge exam packet. I felt like I was back in high school taking the state regents exams. There was no dialogue between the psychologist and us, but her awkward body language and tight jaw showed her discomfort. Jennifer and I exchanged knowing glances and tried to hide our smiles. In a way, sharing our dislike of Dr. Petit helped us deal with the awkwardness of being psychologically evaluated. Dr. Petit clicked her tongue and said, "Read the test and answer each question. You may begin."

"This is ridiculous," Jennifer said under her breath.

It was all I could do not to laugh out loud.

We filled in the little circles of the unending questionnaire until they blurred in front of our eyes.

Question #492 . . . Would you like to be a florist? I started obsessing. Yes, that would be a nice thing to do; no, I don't know if that's a career I want; yes, arranging flowers could be beautiful and creative. *What were they asking?*

"Stephen, I'm not sure how to answer this."

He looked up from the paper, hoping no one noticed me asking him for assistance.

"Liza, you're overthinking this, do you want to be a florist?"

"No."

"That's your answer," he said bluntly.

A lab technician came looking for Jen. She had to give twelve vials of blood. David, Stephen, and I waited in silence in Scot's office. We were all feeling the pressure of the day. Jennifer returned forty-five minutes later. She was ashen and teary-eyed from fatigue and emotion.

Jennifer and Stephen were given a lesson on how to inject, mix, and measure the drugs, just as I had been. They gave her the starter kit of syringes, medicine, and the video. It was seven P.M. when we finally left. We had been there ten hours.

Chapter
24

*S*tephen and David went to have a drink at the restaurant where we would meet them for dinner while Jen and I took a cab to Mom's apartment on Eighty-forth Street and Lexington Avenue. Jennifer collapsed onto the sofa. Usually, she never sat down without inspecting the new sculptures that had begun to clutter the rooms. This evening she was grateful just to close her eyes.

I could tell by my mother's expression and the way she embraced us, looking soft yet severe, that she had something to say. The visit was not solely for a kiss and hug. I sat in the oversize flowered chintz chair opposite my mother and waited while she served us tea. When she began to speak her voice was filled with concern.

"I spoke to Kodie last night. She was so sweet, Jen. She said, 'Nannie, you can't believe how good I'm doing in sculpture.' She said she wants to be a sculptor when she grows up. I told her I'd give her lessons when she comes to New York. She's my grandchild, like Stuart and Sophia." She paused.

"Jen. I'm in a difficult position. You are like my daughter. You are my blood and you've promised a gift to Liza that will complete her life. Yet I'm afraid. I don't like all those drugs. No one knows what the far-reaching consequences will be. I tried to stop Liza, now

I want to stop you both. Liza can adopt. Frankly, I'm against it, only because of the drugs. Your offer showed your love. It was enough." Her voice was forceful.

Jennifer sat up. "Aunt Suzy, the only bad side effect of the drugs is that they'll make me more obnoxious that I am now. Don't be afraid. We've done a lot of research."

My mother obviuosly saw no humor in Jen's words.

"Mom," I interjected, "these are hormones that the body produces naturally."

I understod my mother so well. She knew Laurie would think the idea of carrying my child romantic; she would have done it in a wink. But pointing out the health risk was my mother's responsibility to her sister. I believe her promise to Laurie to take care of Jennifer had priority over my desire to have a baby in this unusual, but most ideal way.

Jennifer rose from the sofa and sat on the chair beside my mother. "Aunt Suzy, Mommy wants me to do this. If she were here she would do it herself. Nothing would stop her. You agree, don't you?"

"Yes, Jen, I know my sister and her boundless enthusiasms. But, if she were here, I would object the same way for the same reasons. We're different people, Laurie and I, and I have to think for both of us. I need time, Jen, and I need to know more about it." They spoke quietly, looking directly and deep into each other's eyes.

I left the room so they could be alone. My mother was in a difficult position. Jennifer was overtired. They had to come to an understanding before we continued. My mother was still the matriarch. She deserved respect.

I came into the room after fifteen minutes. My mother was crying. Jennifer handed her a tissue from her pocket and began to speak. "I don't mean to make you sad. I don't know how you've handled your loss. I've said you're like an ostrich with your head in the sand and don't face reality, but I don't believe it. You are the strong one. I admire you. I know having the baby and giving it to Liza and David will show me that I can go on also. Like you do. Believe me I will be all right. We will all be fine."

My mother nodded. Her voice was firm when she spoke. "Keep

your promise to me, Jennifer. I'm not your mother, but you should know I honestly love you and will care for you."

We had to hurry so as not to be late for dinner; our schedule was tight; later, Jen and Stephen would catch a plane back to Chicago.

"La, Jennifer . . ." My mother stopped us at the door. "You must promise not to put your health in jeopardy; if there is a sign of trouble, you'll stop. Promise you won't put yourself in any long-term emotional or physical danger. I'm not talking about discomfort, that's expected, I'm talking about sickness. This is a promise to me and to Laurie."

Jen kissed her warmly and we both gave her our word. It was an oath between the four of us: my mother, Aunt Laurie, Jen, and me.

We raced off to meet the men at the Carlyle Hotel on Madison Avenue and Seventy-sixth Street, where David and I had gone on our first date. The hotel dining room catered to its customers' desire for quiet and attentive, respectful service. The staff intuited our need for privacy and that made us feel special. The four of us *were* special that night. Beautiful vases of flowers and low lights contributed a warm glow to the elegant unpretentious room and seemed to underscore our feeling of being apart from the rest of society. David and Stephen were already halfway through a bottle of Pinot Grigio. We ordered another with dinner. Jennifer savored every mouthful of the dry white wine like a connoisseur facing a year of exile from civilization. We toasted glass after glass to our having made it through this horrendous day of raw emotion.

"Here's to Jen's bravery."

Jen wrinkled her nose and said solemnly, "To no drinking and no coffee."

"And to the blood tests,"

"And to seeing Scot."

"Here's to Scot."

"To Scot." We all clicked. "This is meant to be."

"To Aunt Laurie."

We were happy and mellow from the wine. Jennifer wasn't sad when she said, "Mommy would be proud of all of us."

"We are lucky she is with us," David said, and refilled our glasses. We clicked again and drank.

I could see Aunt Laurie. She would be sitting between me and Jen, having squeezed every last drop of information on IVF from the doctors and thinking haughtily how powerful we were and perhaps that her sister was too much the skeptic. That would tickle her.

When it was time to go, David and I walked Stephen and Jennifer to the cab. As they drove off, David cried, "It's all so heavy and confusing. So . . . remarkable."

25

*I*n late November of 1996, when our hearts were full of Thanksgiving, I received a message from Joan Petit on my voice mail. We
had been waiting for it. Scot could not legally continue our
gestational-carrier program until the psychologist gave her approval.

She said she thought Jen's MMPI test was invalid because she heard
that Stephen had helped her with the answers. I didn't understand
why the psychologist was telling me this and leaving it as a message
on my answering machine. She had reserved comment as long as possible and now she was obstructing our path. It was as Jennifer had intuitively feared.

I left Dr. Petit a message saying as far as I knew, Stephen gave
his wife no help during the test; if she had a problem, she should
call Jennifer. A week passed; I said nothing to Jen while I waited
for a bomb to be tossed at us, but none came. We never did hear
from Joan Petit again and I never took the time to pursue the matter.
It wasn't important; the psychologist was nothing but one of the
potholes we encountered along our road to childbirth. Scot called
and told me we were scheduled to begin. That's all that mattered.

Mom and Aunt Laurie's mother, our Grandma Reese, lives in a
facility for the elderly. She has her own apartment and socializes

with the other ladies who meet for tea each afternoon. Jennifer told her that she would be pregnant with my baby. It would be Liza's egg and David's sperm.

Grandma Reese said, "Suzy already explained it to me, dear. Some of the girls here think it is indecent." She assumed David and Jen were having sex. IVF was totally beyond her comprehension. I tried and tried to explain the procedure. Eventually she said. "Yes, dear. I understand. That's good." I knew she didn't get it. Her initial interpretation, though, gave Jen and me a good laugh.

David's mother, Frances, called from Florida after she heard the news of our decision. "Liza, is it all right if I send Jennifer something? I hardly know her but I want to let her know that I love her for giving you and David an opportunity to have a child."

She haltingly suggested a pair of diamond drop earrings that had been her mother's, the ones I'd admired when she wore them at our wedding. I hadn't ever heard Frances speak so carefully before. I got the feeling she was afraid she might insult me. It was heartwarming the way she apologized, saying she had wanted me to have the earrings at the birth of David's child. I felt a wave of affection toward her as I glimpsed her devotion to family. Jennifer was almost a stranger to her, but she was trying to treat her with love. I felt that love pass along to me and David as well. Jennifer's gift touched so many people. I wasn't insulted or hurt by Frances' offer. I told her I was honored, and Jennifer would wear the earrings proudly.

Before hanging up, Frances said, "In my generation, when miracles like this occurred, it was only through prayer and godly intervention."

"And today, Frances," I replied, "it would be the same, but for science and Jennifer. It is still a miracle."

Jennifer finally succeeded in reaching her brother. It was Thanksgiving day when Jack called; he said he had been in Los Angeles for six weeks and was relocating his music business and getting an apartment there.

I received a letter from Jennifer. It was clear that when some thought or event was weighing on her, she had begun to explore its meaning by writing and sharing it with me. I was moved and astounded by her openness and willingness to tell me everything. For Jennifer, having the baby was more than a "biological endeavor," and a great gift to me. It was an intellectual and emotional journey.

Dear Liza,

I told Jack about me carrying your baby. He was incredulous and told me the idea was terrible. He thought you and Aunt Suzy would hate me if anything goes wrong. He said I would cause a rift in the family. "Remember how we were blamed for everything in their house?" he said.

I told him Uncle Herbie had called me to thank me for doing this. And we talked about Mommy. Liza, it was the first time your father ever called me. Maybe the only time he really ever spoke to me other than a reprimand. I suppose it's because he always thought of me as a child or a nuisance. Now he admires me. Strangely, that is worth a lot to me, and I told Jack, hoping he would admire me the same way. I wish my brother would understand that having the baby will only do good for everyone. We are a family. We don't all understand each other deeply, but in times of need we are there.

Jack always found fault with me and he was always angry. He said I was doing this to be the center of attention. I suppose he is right, at least from his point of view. Jack was always the difficult one, who was sent away to school, and I remained home close to Mommy and I did get her daily attention. You know, I would have it no other way. I look back to his words and I agree—I was selfish. So now, La, I must scrutinize my motives again. Is it Mommy's attention I long for and am I doing this to win praise? I don't believe this at all. I wish I could convince Jack. He and you are all I have that know all the phases of my life, that knew me as a child with my mother. Jack and I are the only ones that have her living with them alive in their hearts. If I lose Jack, I lose that part of me. There will be no one to recall little nuances or happenings. Yet there has always been a distance between us. We reach out with long arms but don't quite touch.

I wish Jack could be part of this with me. His only reaction was, "It's a big mistake." He said I could be misinterpreting Mommy's message; he said she might have meant for me to bring her light into my life and pass it to Kodie and Austin.

Liza, anything—everything—can be interpreted in hundreds of ways. It is up to each individual to see something and act on it as they themselves see fit; otherwise nothing gets done. I'll be pregnant in January, La, and your baby will be born in October, maybe on my birthday. I think it is time Jack grew up and stopped making me suffer for the past.

Jen

One part in Jennifer's letter stood out for me—the lines about my father. I was surprised she was still affected by him. She had made a point of saying she valued his approval. I wondered if it was not attention, as Jack suspected, but approval she was seeking. I didn't want to bring the subject up to her, but we had a pact of honesty. I didn't want to leave any gray areas in her understanding of her heroic undertaking. I didn't want there to be even the hint of a shadow of misunderstanding to mar the beauty of our connection. Having never been pregnant, it was impossible for me to empathize completely with her, which I tried to do. I called and asked her about her need for approval.

"How can you ask me that?" There was anger in Jennifer's voice, the same anger I'd heard when she predicted Joan Petit's negative assessment. "I told you why. I'm clear on it. You should be, too. If you get hooked looking for trouble, you'll create it. Forget everyone else and their doubts. They come from their own weaknesses and have nothing to do with you and me. Keep the facts straight."

She was adamant and confident and I apologized.

Martin Luber, Jen's father, spoke to her with deep concern about the long-term consequences of being a gestational carrier. He repeated the same question time and again: "Jen, how will you feel when Liza takes the baby or babies to New York City and you won't be able to see or touch or make any decisions about the fruit of your womb?"

Jennifer listened to everyone, but she was as unwavering as a salmon swimming upriver, against the current, determined to create life.

Chapter

26

*J*ennifer was ready to begin Lupron, the drug that would suppress her menstrual cycle so she wouldn't realease her own eggs. Her trial cycle would determine if she was a good candidate for embryo transplant and if she responded favorably to the drugs. On day one of Lupron, she called to say she would let me know when she had received the shot.

I sat down and thought of Jennifer so far away in Chicago, and how close I felt to her. I thought of my IVF cycles and what helped me through them and I thought of three positive things, as Greg prescribed.

OVER THE PAST YEAR, three pigeons had made a nest near the air conditioner outside my bedroom window. The first time I went through IVF, I noticed a bird sitting on an egg. Not surprisingly, this egg became a symbol of my own quest to "hatch" my own egg. I watched that egg every day of my IVF cycle, thinking superstitiously that it represented the egg/embryo in me. As my cycle came to an end, the mother pigeon had disappeared with her egg. One day they were there, the next day they were gone.

The second IVF cycle coincided with the occupation by another mother bird, this time with two eggs. This pigeon would fly off for a while then return to sit on the two eggs. I named them "Fry" and "Licher." As I continued my cycle, she continued hers. This bird disappeared, too, and so did her eggs.

The week before Jen came to New York, I noticed a third bird, this one also sitting on two eggs. I told myself not to get involved this time, but I couldn't help looking out the window at her each day. Two days after Jen left New York, the two eggs hatched. Two tiny baby pigeons were ensconced in the nest on top of the air conditioner. I looked at them every chance I got. I could hear them chirping for their mother. I left water and twigs at the far side of the air conditioner, never touching the nest. The mother bird ignored everything I left her and sat with birdlike dignity on her New York City wire-and-plaster nest. One day I left pieces of bread on the next windowsill; this she took. Twice she flew off, leaving the babies, when she became aware of my presence.

Seeing the birds made me optimistic. They were a fateful sign, a good omen of birth.

Jennifer called half an hour later. "The shot wasn't bad. I feel fine." What was difficult for me, Jennifer made easy.

After three days, I realized Jen was having a hard time on the Lupron. She didn't complain but told me she felt "possessed." She had headaches, just as I'd had, and was moody and emotional. She also had a skin rash. I wished so much I could do something to make it easier for her. I kept offering her a way out. "You've done so much. I'd back out myself. I wouldn't hold it against you."

"La La, you're the one that's feeling remorse. Don't. It's just an ugly pimple. I've had them before and they go away."

"But I know how you hate them."

We both laughed and I sniffed to prevent from crying. Again I thought of the birds I had watched on my windowsill.

One morning I noticed that one of the baby birds looked weak, stretching his little neck and seeming to gasp for breath. I knew something was wrong, as the other bird was alert. When the mother bird returned to the nest she ignored the sick baby. The next morning the baby was dead, tossed from the nest, lying on its back on the air conditioner.

But the remaining baby was thriving. Every day the mother bird took the bread I left for her. In two weeks, he had grown. He had gray-and-black spiky feathers, a classic ugly duckling. His eyes were open. He looked toward me when his mother was gone. I whispered to him softly so he would get used to my voice and not be afraid. It made me happy to watch his growth, but it also gave me a pang of jealousy to think what might have been for me. The weather was very cold. I worried that the baby might fall off the air conditioner, what with the wind and rain. I tried to think of something to put out to protect him, but came up with nothing. I kept trying to be positive, telling myself not to interpret any mishap the baby bird suffered as bad tidings for me.

Watching the lives of these birds showed me how, in nature, only the strong survive. It didn't matter who you were. My attitudes and expectations were meaningless.

The second night Jen was on the medication, she called me frantically at the restaurant. She said she didn't have enough Lupron to fill the syringe. I told her that couldn't be possible. I knew the starter kit supplied enough for two weeks of shots. She insisted it was true. Clearly, something was wrong. Jennifer put a call in to the hospital, but at ten P.M. nobody was there.

A few minutes later, she called me back. She said she realized she had mistakenly used the wrong syringe, the huge one that was for the progesterone. Somehow it had been put into the same bag as the Lupron syringes.

"La, I feel so stupid and embarrassed. Do you think I'll screw everything up?"

She was so concerned about me and I was scared and nervous only for her. "Why are you even doing this?" I asked. "Throw all this stuff away and forget about it." I didn't want her to feel trapped.

"No, I'm fine, I don't want you to think I'm stupid. I pray I didn't

mess up the cycle. Am I going to die with this overdose in my body?"
She had taken ten times the prescribed dosage.

I called the emergency room at Cornell; the doctor said the overdose would do no harm. He suggested that we call our specialist in
the morning to see if any future doses would need readjusting.

I called Jen back right away.

Again, she amazed me. She had just taken an overdose of a powerful and possibly dangerous drug and all that concerned her was our
cycle. I was worried about Jennifer. I promised to keep her healthy.

Before beginning the cycle of a gestational carrier, the law requires
all parties involved to sign a contract. David was in contact with a
lawyer, in Chicago, Terry Fuerst, whose practice was limited to cases
involving infertility, surrogacy, and adoption.

The contract covered any eventuality: should Jen get pregnant and
not want to give up the baby, should the fetus be unhealthy and
have to be aborted, should David and I change our minds. It was
strange to make these provisions for events that hadn't yet happened, but it was necessary. The contract looked fine to me and
David except that it did not give us enough responsibility for com-
pensation should Jennifer become disabled in any way as a result of
the pregnancy. Patricia Greene suggested that we take out a disability insurance plan for Jennifer, and we did so, for our own piece
of mind. We were proceeding with great caution, for the unknown
was always there, lurking.

Jennifer had started the estrogen patches and was doing better. She
was bothered by the skin rash and itching, but she learned to alter-
nate the patches between her buttocks and her abdomen, thereby
allowing for the surrounding area to heal. At the end of the month,
it was time to test the preparatory cycle to see if her uterus had
responded to the estrogen and progesterone and would accept the
transferred embryos.

Jennifer's doctor in Chicago, Isabel Isola, was a slim woman in
her mid-thirties, with a girlish appearance and long dark hair. She
always wore a clinician's coat over her skirt and blouse. Confident

and capable, she understood Jennifer's specific IVF treatments and related to her emotionally, trying to make everything as easy for her as she could. She knew Jennifer's work schedule and never made her wait for an appointment. The entire staff was considerate and like a team they cheered us on. Each morning at eight o'clock before going to work, Jennifer arrived for her tests and was given a glass of fresh orange juice. "Energy," they said. On this icy morning in December, the endometrial biopsy, to determine whether she could nourish the embryos, was scheduled. Jennifer wasn't afraid. She trusted Dr. Isola. The doctor took her hand.

"Jennifer. It may be painful for a moment. I'll be quick; afterward there is no lingering pain. Are you all right?"

"I'm fine," Jennifer replied. "Stephen will take me home after. I'm not going to work today."

I was sorry I wasn't in Chicago to go with her. Neither of us had undergone this procedure and didn't know what to expect. Jennifer called me from her bedroom at home. Her voice was tight and controlled. I knew she was in pain.

"It hurt tremendously. It was the first time I questioned out loud why I was doing this. La, I really hollered and it wasn't nice. They put this device, similar to a hole puncher, inside of me and took out an inch-long cylinder-shaped sample of flesh that looked like a fat earthworm. I could feel the tissues being cut from my insides."

Knowing she was enduring this pain for me made me suffer almost as she did. I hadn't known the procedure would hurt so badly, and even after Jen's pain eased, mine continued. It wasn't guilt. Jen and I had discussed that. We both understood we had made educated choices. It was something more, the helplessness you feel when you see someone you love suffer. It was frustration and anger. It was feeling inadequate next to Jen's bravery and wanting to give an equal gift in return and wondering if I could. How does someone handle such kindness and self-sacrifice.

I always believed that if I had to make a choice, I would choose correctly if I was able to judge the options honestly. It was difficult for me to judge in this case. Was it selfish for me to do another IVF cycle with Jennifer as the gestational carrier? Was I not creating unforseen problems for Jennifer and her family. How would she explain to six-year-old Dakota that the baby in her belly was Aunt Liza's and wouldn't be her brother or sister? What would Stephen tell people: "My wife is pregnant—no, it's not my child"? How would all this affect their healing marriage? How does a man give up intimacy with his mate and watch a baby grow inside her knowing it isn't his? Stephen becomes the victim. This birth is a mission for me, David and Jen. Her husband is a soldier to have joined our corps.

In retrospect, I didn't think Jennifer and I had always been as close as we should have to undertake such an extreme mission together. There were years of separation while I was in Spain, but our love had a strong foundation. Perhaps it was because of the role models set by our mothers, and the value they always placed on family togetherness. The sisters, together, had somehow managed to transcend hardships to make life joyful.

Jennifer and I talked and she told me she could continue our project as long as she knew she wouldn't have to undergo another endometrial biopsy. I promised her she'd never have to because I wouldn't let her. Jennifer was unable to gauge her own strength. I felt pride in and gratitude for who she was.

I faxed Dr. Isola a letter, thanking her for being so helpful, supportive, and kind to Jennifer. *It makes things easier for all of us,* I wrote. *I am proud of my cousin's strength. I brag about her to anyone who will listen. Her perseverance amazes me. I trust Jennifer with my baby and I trust you, Dr. Isola. Again, I thank you for your kindness to all of us.* Dr. Isola had renewed my faith that there was also humanity in the medical establishment.

When I spoke to Scot the next day he assured me that Jennifer didn't need to have another endometrial-lining biopsy before the transfer; the test proved the lining was as lush and thick as Jennifer had predicted. The progesterone had thickened the lining, rendering her as a good candidate for accepting the embryos.

*A*s I said before, Jennifer and I considered ourselves pioneers. The only real difference in our view of our adventure was in the way each of us referred to the birth. Jennifer would always say "when the baby is born." And I couldn't help but say "*if* the baby is born." Perhaps I used the word "if" to protect myself from the terrible disappointment that failure would bring.

I tried continually to play Greg's mind trick, concentrating on three thoughts that would make me happy. It helped me. On the whole, I was more optimistic than pessimistic.

The baby bird outside my window had gotten so big; he had learned to spread his wings. While I was adjusting the curtains one day, the baby faced me and pumped out his chest and strutted as if to protect his turf and frighten me away—such a tough little guy for someone who was only an egg three weeks earlier. The mother hovered over him. It looked like she was biting him and I was about to knock on the window to scare her away when I realized she was putting the food I had left into the baby's mouth. The mother regurgitated chewed-up Jewish rye bread and fed it to her offspring. Within a few days, I could see the baby bird flapping its wings and getting ready to fly. I didn't want him to leave.

On Christmas Eve, I took my first home ovulation test. A drop of urine turned the patch pink, indicating that I was ovulating. On the third day of my menstrual period, Jen and I were scheduled to begin our cycle together. It would be the first day of 1997, the New Year, and I would start Lupron. Jennifer had been on the drug since the test cyle. Her body was in a state of medically induced menopause, the hormones preventing her from releasing her own eggs.

At the end of this cycle, Jennifer could become pregnant. I felt positive about this.

I also had the first shot of Lovenox on January 1 instead of heparin. Scot and the hematologist prescribed Lovenox, which is also a blood thinner but less devastating than the heparin I had taken during my previous IVF attempts. David gave me the shot in my right arm, and aside from a slight burning, I felt well all day. We had been at our house on Long Island for the past ten days. It was a rare restful period, going to dinner parties and being with friends, and I had been in a holiday frame of mind. As we drove back to New York City, I rested my head against the seat back, happily believing for the first time that David and I had a good chance of having a child and a new life this new year.

January was to be filled with injections, often five a day. Daily visits to the hospital for blood tests and sonograms, all a repetition of my previous IVF attempts; however, now the pain would be doubled, since I would suffer Jennifer's as well as my own. By the end of the month, we would have endured the anxiety of egg development, retrieval, David's surgery, and the embryo transfer. These medical procedures were exhausting, but most daunting would be the changes this year would ring in our lives. Forever and ever I would be in a state of beautiful indebtedness to my cousin.

I no longer had coffee in the morning, nor would I until the baby was born. If Jennifer could give up coffee, I told myself, so could I; and if she could be so positive, so could I; we each had so much to gain.

Jen called late at night to tell me that she had several pimples on her face as a result of the progesterone she had taken the previous month during the trial cycle and that she "hated me." We laughed, but she was upset about her skin. As if a pimple could mar such beauty as hers.

January 1, 1997—from Jennifer's journal

The sun woke me early this morning. I was reluctant to leave my lovely dream of floating colors. I didn't hear Austin come in. "Snuggle me, Mama, it's cold in here," he murmured as he climbed in bed beside me. I picked up the heavy quilt I had thrown onto the floor during the night and covered him. "I was watching you sleep," my son said as I kissed his neck, breathing in the warm fragrance of his youth. "Mama, are you up?"

"I'm up. Is Daddy in the bathroom?"

"No, I think he's out. Kodie is making breakfast for us. I will tell her you're ready." He hopped off the bed and called downstairs, "Kodie, she's up!"

I stretched, loving the family about me. I heard the dishes being moved in the kitchen, then Dakota's cautious footsteps ascending the stairs. I sat up and brushed out my hair that had matted to my head from a night of profuse sweating. Each night is a battle with my body temperature, since I began the Lupron. I sleep uncovered in a skimpy nightgown, while Stephen is piled high with blankets. Usually, Kodie and Austin won't come into the bedroom—it is too cold. In the Windy City, to sleep with the window wide open during the winter is to expect icicles on the radiator by morning. Many nights Stephen gets up and sleeps in the twin bed in Kodie's room.

Kodie came in and placed the tray on my lap.

"Where's Daddy?" I asked.

"He went out early. Is he mad? He looked mad at me."

"He's not mad at you, Kodie. Daddy didn't sleep well, that's all." I looked at the black cocktail dress I was planning to wear last night still spread across the chaise. It was the one I wore

three years ago after giving birth to Austin. Now I have already gained ten pounds, just from the drugs. New Year's Eve—I slept through it. I had meant to get up from my nap and dress for the late dinner party we were invited to at the home of Stephen's business associate. Stephen wanted to go to that party and yet he wouldn't wake me. I am so tired lately. The drugs still in my body from that last cycle make me feel exhausted even before my day at the office begins. On the weekends I have no energy or interest in anything but sleep.

There is tension between Stephen and me since the preparatory cycle began last month. In bed last night I felt him fondling my breast and rubbing, so very gently, the secret spot at the small of my back that never failed to arouse me. I found it annoying. I was so tired; I turned my back and, without further ado, fell asleep. I don't know if Stephen slept or if he got up and went downstairs for ice cream or to go through his sports magazines as he often does when he is upset. This morning he must have left early so that he wouldn't have to confront me or feel guilty. All week I have been falling asleep after helping Kodie with her homework and tucking Austin in bed, leaving my husband alone. He never says a word, but I can read his face and know he is feeling left out, and unneeded, which isn't true. I need him more than ever in case I slacken. Since we're back together, after our separation, we scrutinize each other for signs of weakness, of returning to the frame of mind that caused the rift: noncommunication, and lack of trust in our love. When we finish this and he is beside me, it will make our marriage an impenetrable fortress because we will have done it together. I feel strongly about this and have told him, hoping he will recognize our mutual need.

Stephen and I always had an active sex life. Lovemaking was an important part of our marriage, for pleasure and security, even when I was pregnant with Kodie and Austin. Now, when he desires it and needs it the most, I refuse him.

I don't feel guilty. To pass my mother's light to Liza is my priority. I do feel sorry, though. We have only had sex twice since I began the Lupron thirty days ago. My head wants to, but my body won't respond. Neither have I been a good companion—Stephen comes home from work, we have dinner, and I go upstairs with the kids, then I go to sleep, after he gives me the injection. He gives it to me each night, and if I'm asleep he nudges me awake, injects, and I fall back asleep, glad that I spent time with Dakota and Austin and their special needs. I miss them when I'm at work. I don't want to lose a day of their childhood, not for my husband, Liza, or the baby; Kodie and Austin can't be deprived of their mother because of this.

Stephen came upstairs and finally we talked.

I put my arms out to my husband. "I'm so sorry about last night. I know you wanted to go to the party."

He sat on the bed and embraced me. Then he stood up, so tall, looking down at me in the bed. "Jen, we have no life anymore. No life of any kind."

"I know. David and Liza are going through the same thing; the drugs will be over soon, after I'm pregnant."

"Liza and David will be going about their lives, working, taking vacations, loving—you know what I mean. I miss my wife. We have nine months more of this. They're free to do whatever they like. It's not the same."

"I'll be over this tiredness after I stop the drugs and am pregnant. You remember how I was before Dakota and Austin were born. We went out dancing, bike riding—everything. I was fine during my pregnancies."

"Jen. You can still change your mind."

"Stephen. Please. I'm going to do it."

He went to the door. There's no talking to me once my mind is made up. That well he knew his wife. "I'll watch the kids while you shower," he said with finality.

"Stephen. We've gone over this again and again. I'll be a better person after; you'll like me better. I know you love me, but you'll like me better. I promise."

"I'll be downstairs." He went into the hallway.

"Stephen."

He turned and came back to the bed. "Jen. I believe you
think this will work. I know the pain you're in since Laurie's
death. I love you and I'll do whatever I can to help you have
a happy life for the kids and for me. I support you one hundred
percent. Just be sure, now, before you have a baby inside you,
that it's what you want, and if it will be the answer. I don't
doubt that you can do it. Just make sure you won't cause
yourself more pain."

"What do you mean, more pain?"

"I mean giving up the baby."

"It's Liza's baby, Stephen. I'm miserable now. How many
ways have I tried to get better? This is meant to be. I know it
is right. And, Stephen, I thank you with all my heart for
understanding."

"I'll wait for you downstairs. We'll do a barbecue tonight.
The girls will help me. Take it easy. But once more—think
hard."

. . . I will work this out with Stephen. I believe his commitment
to be my partner in this program. In just a short time the hard,
crazy-headed part will be over. I will feel better after the drugs,
when I am pregnant. I felt special and flirtatious during my
other pregnancies. I was fun to be with. I will be the same very
soon—after the drugs. Liza is going to have her baby; nothing
is going to stand in our way. I survived the endometrical-lining
biopsy, that was the worst. Scot said that was the only painful
part, and he promised I don't have to have that again.
Childbearing, even a cesarean birth, which I know I won't
have, is a picnic compared to that. Just as I willed Austin to
be born vaginally, so will I with Liza's baby.

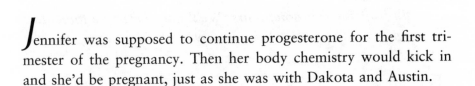

*J*ennifer was supposed to continue progesterone for the first trimester of the pregnancy. Then her body chemistry would kick in
and she'd be pregnant, just as she was with Dakota and Austin.

On the first day of her progesterone injection, she called. "Talk
us through finding the spot again," she said. Stephen was on the
extension. "We've read and reread the manual and watched the
video, but when the reality of plunging that dagger of a needle in
the flesh of your beloved is upon you, it's terrifying."

I knew the routine. "Ready? Standing up . . . put your hands on
your hipbones, your thumbs to the back."

"Okay."

"Now, let Stephen wipe it well with alcohol."

"Yes. Okay."

"Take a pinch, right where your thumb is, that's the correct
spot."

"Got it, we'll call you when it's over."

I hung up, feeling sick, nervous, and upset. Jennifer was brave
and said she wasn't frightened, but I hated the pain David and I
were causing her. David went into the outer hallway to smoke a
cigarette, which is something he rarely does. I hadn't seen him leave

and called him to sit by the phone next to me. When he returned, I said, "This is going to be a tough year."

After a few minutes that seemed like an hour Jennifer called again. Her voice was light, I thought she was smiling. "I'm fine, La. It burned but not as much as I thought it would. I'm glad we called you about the position. You and David are experts. Stephen was more shaken than I was, but he was very strong, as usual."

"Jen, when are you going to tell Kodie and Austin?" I asked.

"Liza, when I'm truly pregnant. At that time, I'll explain to them so they understand from the beginning that the baby growing in their mother's tummy will not be their sister or brother, and it won't be living at home with us. Mommy won't bring a baby home from the hospital. The baby will go home with Aunt La and Uncle David and I am very happy to help them have their baby. After all, I have the two best children possible and that is all we want."

"What will you do if the pregnancy test is negative?" I heard Stephen ask.

"There is no possibility. I love you all. Good night."

The next day was day two of Lovenox for me. David offered to give me the shot before he went to work, but I wanted to do it myself in case he had to go away on business during the cycle. I tried it in my left thigh. I forgot how tough the skin is and the needle didn't go through. David had a practiced flick-of-the-wrist action that I tried to imitate. This time it went in. It didn't sting as much as it did in my arm, but the area was swollen and I could see it turning black and blue with a hard red welt. If Jennifer can do it, so can I, I told myself.

That day Jennifer went to Dr. Isola for her blood test and sonogram. Her uterus had thickened and the doctor told her she was responding to the medicines the way they had hoped. Step-by-step, everything was going well. Jen was especially cheerful that her complexion was clearing up even though her butt was polka-dotted with marks from the estrogen patches.

I recorded the updates on my friends who were going through in vitro.

Hanna had the amnio test and is pregnant with healthy twins—a boy and a girl. She is in her fourth month and beginning to thicken at the waist. She's already wearing maternity clothes. Hanna had four failed IVF cycles.

Allison is the daughter-in-law of a close friend of my mother's who introduced us when they came to Sambuca for dinner. At the time we were both on our first IVF cycle and needed an ally against the depression caused by Lupron. We became friends. Allison is my age. She had one failed IVF cycle and gave birth to a daughter after the second attempt. Today she is three months along in a pregnancy that resulted naturally.

Mindy: The doctors found some scarring and recommended that she have another procedure. She is very secretive, so I don't know what caused the scarring or what procedure has been recommended. Her condition is very different from mine. Her problem is with her reproductive organs; mine is blood-related.

Stephanie is still trying. This will be IVF cycle number four. She would love to be pregnant at the same time as Jennifer and me.

It was January 3 and day three of Lupron. I did the Lovenox in my left arm. This blood thinner still burned and the injection site bled for fifteen minutes. I called the hematologist at Cornell. He said the Lovenox shouldn't create a problem, and prevent normal clotting. I probably hit a blood vessel. He suggested not putting the needle all the way in; the syringes, he said, were designed for people a lot fleshier then I was. That made me absurdly happy: he thought of me as thin.

I finally spoke to Dr. Marle after leaving six messages. He is one of the IVF doctors at Cornell whom Jen and I met when we had our first consultation with Scot. At that time, we asked him how many embryos would be transferred into Jennifer's uterus. He said three was usually the maximum, in order to reduce the risk of multiple births. Because he was so highly regarded—the IVF doctors at Cornell considered him the leading specialist on this subject—I wanted to ask him about "selective reduction," the procedure that is performed should all three embryos adhere to the uterus and continue to grow, which would result in the birth of triplets. In such an event, what potential risk was there to Jennifer and the remaining fetus(es)? We all had discussed the medical, financial, and emotional complications that carrying triplets would entail.

"Mrs. Freilicher, I'm not at ease discussing this with you," the doctor answered. "I don't want to be responsible for your making a decision based on my advice."

His blunt lack of sympathy took me aback. "I'm not asking you to get involved," I quickly explained. "I understand the decision is ours. I'm merely asking for information, for knowledge based on your experience. I would like you to help us understand selective reduction so we can act with intelligence should it become an option."

"Your lawyer can give you the information you need," he said tersely.

"Why should this come from a lawyer? I want medical advice. It isn't a legal matter."

"I'll give you the names and numbers of other doctors. There's a good man at Mount Sinai—"

I interrupted. "I refuse to speak to anyone there."

"Well, then, Mrs. Freilicher, speak to your lawyer."

He didn't say "good luck" or "sorry I couldn't be more helpful." We've all met cold, uncaring doctors. I wonder when they develop such attitudes, if they are a defense mechanism to distance themselves from the suffering of their patients. I, unlike David, have a problem with such doctors.

I couldn't understand why Dr. Marle, a specialist in the field, wouldn't discuss selective reduction with us, but after my initial annoyance passed, I assumed he was merely protecting himself.

I called Jennifer.

"I have the name of a doctor in Chicago," she told me. "Dr. Isola gave it to me. She said this man can answer our questions."

"Jen, it was our agreement. The bottom line is you make the decision where your body is concerned. Remember that. You decide.

If you want to carry one fetus and reduce the others, it's your decision."

Jennifer didn't want to carry triplets, and I couldn't blame her, but it wasn't so simple. "How can I choose to eliminate one or two embryos clinging to my body for life? Which ones?" she asked. This was a no-win situation. We were transferring three embryos, praying that they would adhere to the uterus and cell division would continue, and yet in the same prayer we hoped not to have to make the decision to terminate life. Ultimately, this would be Jennifer's decision.

Lately, the baby bird has been hanging out on the edge of the air conditioner. I turned up the heat; my radiator is below the air conditioner and I hoped it would warm the unit. Yesterday, I dropped some bread-and-cracker mixture soaked in milk on the a/c to see if the baby would eat it himself. I have been leaving this mixture for the mother also, but a few other birds discovered the food and tried to carry it away or eat it. The baby opens his beak as if he expects to be fed by those birds. Perhaps he thinks one of them is his mother. They push him aside. Eventually the birds flew away, I think because the baby was too annoying. He is about six weeks old and quite big. As I watched him, he started flapping his wings. For a split second I thought he was going to fall off the air conditioner, but then he flew upward. His wings made a loud whooshing sound and then he was in the air. I was cheering out loud. He looked a bit uncoordinated, but he was flying. He flew up two floors and then his mother flew beside him and touched him with her wings as if to guide him. They landed on a nearby windowsill. I felt privileged, as if he had waited for me so I would see his first flight. Right before my eyes, my little baby bird, who couldn't eat on his own, had opened his wings and begun to fly.

*D*avid and I were on a plane headed for Chicago. New York Hospital Cornell Medical Center required that we sign a contract before they would transfer the embryos to the gestational carrier.

Patricia had referred us to Terry Fuerst, our Chicago attorney. The meeting would be between Fuerst, representing David and me, and the Scheus' lawyer. None of us would be present. The contract was intended to provide a clear picture of David and my legal and moral responsibilities to Jennifer and Stephen before, during, and after the pregnancy. According to the contract, if there were to be any risk whatsoever to Jennifer's health or life, the pregnancy would be terminated. Jennifer's mental and physical well-being were pre-eminent. If the fetus should develop a disease, Down's syndrome, or suffer a birth defect, Jennifer, as well as David and I, could elect to have an abortion. Also, Jennifer would be the one to make any decisions regarding selective reduction. The contract also covered our full financial obligation for all medical and other expenses incurred during the pregnancy.

Jennifer and Stephen's obligations to us were also stipulated. Jennifer was bound to care for her health and to protect the fetus from disease or trauma. She agreed not to drink alcoholic beverages, not to smoke, and not to drink coffee. As a couple, to ensure that no disease would be transmitted to the fetus, they were to use condoms during sex and promise not to have extramarital partners.

At the time of birth, David and I would witness the delivery. The infant would be laid on Jennifer's stomach and David would cut the umbilical cord. I would be the first to hold the baby, then David, then Jennifer, who would not nurse the infant. If the child should be a boy, the circumcision would be done in New York by a moil. It would be a bris, according to the Jewish faith of the baby's parents—me and David.

The contract initiated a paper trail establishing our maternity and paternity for our biological baby. This was very important to document and would be required at the time of adoption in the Illinois court system. We knew that according to Illinois law, we would have to adopt the baby. After the birth, we would appear in court before going home to sign the legal adoption papers.

We also agreed to bring the baby or babies to Jennifer's house before returning to New York so her children, and Stephen's daughters, could see their cousin.

This issue was of special importance and had to be handled with great sensitivity. Kodie and Austin deserved to see the baby that they had made room for in their lives, whom they related to, as did Jennifer, with tenderness, and whom they would learn to care for. They also had to see David and me as the parents of the infant. We had to remove any idea of a threat that their mother would give them away. Though Stephen's daughters were old enough to reason with, we had to make sure they, too, had no doubts of their family security.

I knew the contract would bring relief to Jennifer and Stephen. Often, I imagine, questions arose in their minds that they felt would be insulting to ask us. With everything in black and white, Jennifer need have no doubts about her safety.

I hoped all four of us would emerge from this legal business unscathed. We didn't foresee a storm on the horizon, but where emotions are involved, no one knows where or when the lightning bolts will strike.

• • •

I was looking forward to seeing Jennifer, Stephen, and the kids; it had been so long. Austin must be a big boy now, I thought. I wished I didn't mind flying so much, because when Jen was pregnant, we'd be coming to Chicago often.

I finally met Christine, the French au pair who lived with Jennifer and watched Kodie and Austin. She had long blond hair like Jennifer and considered her a friend and mentor. She loved the children and had become an important part of Jennifer's family. Christine's dedication gave Jennifer peace of mind during her long day away from home. Christine and I had established an ongoing telephone relationship, and I admit that I often plagued her with questions about Jennifer's frame of mind. I was afraid if Jen was overexhausted she wouldn't tell me. I was glad Christine would be there with Jen after the birth.

During our visit, Jennifer did not sit down for a minute. I thought she'd be tired out from Kodie and Austin's endless demands and by Alexis and Devan, Stephen's daughters, who spent most weekends with them. But Jennifer seemed to be energized by the nonstop pace of motherhood.

At last, on Saturday evening, we left all four kids home with Christine and dined at Jennifer's favorite Italian restaurant, Antonio's, a former coffeehouse across from the old train station in Lake Forest. At least "coffeehouse" is what it was discreetly called back in the days when Chicago was more renowned for its underground organizations. The place was now owned by the third-generation Antonio, who ran it almost like a private club, handpicking reservations for his dozen tables. The bartender, Giro, and the waiters, Paul and Sket, knew Stephen and Jennifer, and made a big fuss when we came in. There was a lot of cheek-to-cheek kissing that reminded me of my time in Spain. Jennifer was greeted similarly by a few colorful characters at the bar who dated back to the proprietorship of Antonio I. Jennifer said she couldn't remember a time when they were not there. I felt their eyes frisk me from head to toe as we passed to our booth in the rear. Almost instantly Antonio sent over an antipasto. I laughed to myself; the restaurant business was the same all over the world—a lot of showbiz and hospitality. And mustachioed Antonio played the role with a twinkle in his eye. Stephen put change in the old-fashioned jukebox, which was probably of the same vintage as the tin ceiling. A moment later, Frank Sinatra's voice boomed out "My Way." How apropos for us, I remember thinking. We were doing it *our* way.

We reminisced and laughed about the path we'd taken and the people we had met and obstacles some had put out in an effort to change our minds. I could see how excited Jennifer was. We were nearing transfer. She looked radiant, not tired, as I had expected, what with her hectic schedule. Jennifer still got up each workday morning at five-thirty to blow-dry her hair and put on makeup before leaving the house. She was always beautiful.

We hadn't met Terry Fuerst but only spoken to her on the telephone. She had been compassionate and efficient and confided in us that she herself had gone through IVF twice and eventually adopted a little girl. Made confident by Patricia's reference, David and I expected the two lawyers would write up a contract that would be agreeable to us all.

We arrived in New York around seven-thirty on Sunday evening and I had time to get to Sambuca to bid good night to the late-night dinner crowd. David and I then sat down to plate of pasta. I was keeping to my vow of no wine. We both felt peaceful about having settled the contract issue. Jennifer knew she was cared for and we had lifted what Stephen might have feared would become his financial burden.

So, why, when the phone rang the next day, was Jennifer's voice so irate?

Chapter
30

*J*ennifer's job was to negotiate contracts for television stations to air commercials. A would-be buyer would call her and explain their requirements. For instance, Post cereal wanted to air their commercials from March 2 through April 12. The bid would be given to all stations, including the independent ones. Jennifer's job was to get the commercial contracts for her stations.

She prided herself on her keen business sense and accurate memory. Each negotiation involved a multitude of detail. Unfortunately, since she began the Lupron in December, she found she was becoming forgetful. It made her fear she would lose her competitive edge in her cutthroat world.

January 6, 1997

I am well aware that in an office atmosphere I can't selfishly be a prima donna because of my personal pursuits. Fellow workers resent it, and because IVF, in itself, is so controversial, I don't want anyone asking me, "Why should you play God?" IVF, though not as well known as abortion, receives the same hysterical reaction from the same fanatics. When I begin to show, I will merely say, "I am pregnant."

In my office I am able to see, on a small scale, what has prevailed throughout the world. People are judgmental of others. Individuals measure themselves against the people around them and are often quick to find fault, criticize, and be destructive if they feel the one they are judging has an advantage. History proves it. If I let it be known that I am a gestational carrier, the women in the office would regard me with some awe and much disapproval. I would be a threat to them as women. The men, in my opinion, would be emasculated. I was a threat. I am a woman who can have a child without a man. Women are supposed to need a man. To be able to achieve the ultimate—a child, without a man? Not acceptable. And for that same woman to be earning more money than many of them and have the authority to overrule their business decisions—it would not sit favorably with those men and women with poor self-esteem. My being a gestational carrier, my own decision, is too much for these people, so I'll keep it a secret.

Only my assistant, Ellen, knows what I am doing. I have trusted her with the truth and I rely on her to remind me of schedules. I can't make excuses for my forgetfulness and expect to be pardoned by those who are only waiting to slit my throat.

I keep slips of paper in my personal organizer to remind me of my position at the bargaining table. Because of the drugs and how they keep me disoriented, I often get lost in the negotiations and am unable to follow what is being said. This could be a calamity for the station, as large sums of money are at stake, and it could also cost me a great deal in commissions if I make an error and lose a deal.

I have notes on when to take each injection and when to change the estrogen patches, when to go for my blood tests and sonograms. I have grocery lists to give Christine and reminders of Kodie's or Austin's checkups at the pediatrician or dentist. I keep notes on when Austin or Kodie needs new shoes. Their feet grow quickly.

Liza warned me that Lupron created feelings of doom. I didn't know about the forgetfulness, but then Dr. Isola explained to me that people react differently to drugs. I wasn't in a state of depression before I began the drug, but if I lose my job it would be the beginning of financial doom for Stephen and me.

When I returned from lunch today, Kathy O'Brien, one of the IVF nurses at Cornell who works closely with Scot in the gestational-carrier program, called to tell me that I needed to have a cervical culture and specific blood workups to ascertain if there was any infection in the mucous seal of my uterus. She said she needed the test done today and have the results faxed to her as soon as they were in.

My immediate thought was I had overlooked something. I had been to Dr. Isola this morning. Surely, if there was a pertinent test she would have been informed and done it. I checked my schedule—no mention of the test. I called Dr. Isola. She had no knowledge of it. When I called Kathy she very coolly said . . . she forgot. Forgot! Now I have to find a way to leave work and drive to the doctor's office without causing too much attention. I'm tired. Why couldn't she have at least called Dr. Isola this morning when she knew I was there? She even had an hour extra to think about it because of the time difference in New York. I have double-checked not to overlook any of my obligations. She's not on Lupron. What's her excuse?

Now that I've blown off some steam by writing this journal entry, I'll call Liza.

I was in my office at the restaurant. The phone was busy. We are usually quiet the week after the holiday parties, but perhaps because of the recent spell of mild weather, people were still eager to go out for an evening.

"Liza." It was Jennifer, and I knew from her breathless tone that something bad had happened. I always worry about her. Maybe she was hurt in an accident or sick, I immediately thought.

"What? What, Jen?"

"That Kathy is not on the ball." She told me what had happened.

I was as angry as she was. "If she forgot this, what else has she forgotten?"

"Exactly."

"We have to call Scot right away. Maybe she made a mistake. If you needed these tests, I think Dr. Isola would have been informed. I'll call Scot and get back to you at the office with a conference call. He'll tell us."

"No, I can't wait. I have to get to Dr. Isola before she leaves the office. We have to get that test done, even if Kathy made a mistake. I'm leaving now. I'll just say I'm sick. Damn. If Kathy were within range, I know I would murder her." She hung up.

I called Scot's office, hoping the three of us could talk together right away. His secretary said he would call back in half an hour— he was with a patient. Jennifer, who was inundated with work at her office, said she could wait only half an hour. Half an hour later Scot's secretary called me.

"Dr. Gorin is unable to call you until after six o'clock tonight."

"You said half an hour—Jennifer and I rearranged our schedules to get that call. A very important test hinges on this call. I must speak to him. Can't you understand the importance of this? I must speak to him now!" I could feel my frustration and anger growing.

"Well, Dr. Gorin has a business to run and he can't call you before then."

She said that to the wrong person. "Listen to me, both Jennifer and I have businesses to run as well, and just because he's a doctor doesn't mean his business is more important than ours." I was outraged. "This can't wait."

"He'll call you later," she said, unruffled by my outburst.

"The biggest problem is that doctors can get away with that kind of disregard because they know we need them."

"He will call you back. This is not an emergency. What doctor do you know who returns a patient's call in half an hour?"

"This is an emergency. Our cycle could fail."

"I'll have him call you," she said, and hung up.

I slammed down the phone. There was nothing to do but wait. I called Jennifer. She said she was going to the doctor immediately. We didn't say anything else. I could sense her fear as she could sense mine. *I forgot.* Was all we had done to be ruined by one person's faulty memory? Each phase of this program was so precisely timed. We couldn't afford to be blindsided by sloppy detail work. It was awful to have to depend on other people.

It was well after six o'clock when Scot finally called. I insisted he read my chart, but he said no one else was in the office to get it and he'd do it himself first thing in the morning.

"Scot, Kathy said those tests should have been done today and no one knew about it: neither Jennifer nor Dr. Isola. Kathy is making mistakes that could ruin us. We need to know tonight. I can't waste another day. I'll hold on. Please. Find the chart." I was trying hard to contain myself, but he read my message of anger and urgency loud and clear.

I heard him opening and closing drawers, then he noisily picked up the telephone. "Liza, I don't see the results of your day-three bloods and cultures," he said with surprise.

"I did them two months ago!"

"They have to be done again."

"That's the problem," I began in exasperation. "No one is on top of things."

"I have to study this, Liza. I'll call Jennifer. Maybe I can still get her at the doctor's office. If I miss her I'll get her at home." He hung up curtly.

I couldn't concentrate on my work at the restaurant after that. I just sat and waited. Jennifer called me an hour and a half later from Dr. Isola's office. The doctor had done the test. Scot called as she was about to leave. He said Kathy read the chart incorrectly, the tests had actually been requested for the following day.

"But still," Jennifer said, her voice tired but angry, "Dr. Isola had no request for the culture or the blood workups. If we didn't check on Kathy, this would have been overlooked. Kathy! I'm glad it was a test and not a medicine she told us to take or not take. Our bodies are on a time clock, you know. The reproductive cycle doesn't wait and give us another chance. An error can put an end to this cycle."

"It seems no one at the center is monitoring the details of our schedules," I said, not meaning to make an already bad situation worse. "I guess we wrongfully assumed that because Scot is a friend, he'd have a personal interest and not treat us like just another case, another day at the office. Besides, if our case fails, it would be Dr. Scot Gorin's failure—not Kathy's. What's the matter with people?"

Jen and I were silent on the phone. Then she said in her optimistic voice, "Well, we're fine so far, Lollipop. We did the test, that's what counts. I bet Scot will speak to me again. He always plays Mr. Nice Guy with me; it goes back to high school. People don't change."

Jennifer called me again as I was turning out the lights at Sambuca and ready to close the restaurant. This time she was laughing. "Mr. Nice Guy called as I predicted. Listen to the conversation."

" 'Jen,' he said to me in a butter-would-melt-in-his-mouth voice. 'I admit I didn't know where either of you were in your cycle. I had depended on Kathy. I didn't know you'd had the endometrial biopsy until I studied your chart. I had given Kathy the schedule and expected her to synchronize all details and tell me your progress. I am glad you and Liza caught me on this.'

" 'Scot,' I said to him. 'This program is new, you said so yourself. How could you give Kathy that responsibility? She's had no experience; she's not qualified. This is a frightening situation.'

"His answer was, 'I've no excuse. All I can say is I promise to myself, to you, and to Liza and all my patients, it will not happen again. I thank God it was only a small blunder.'

"I kept my voice firm. 'Check through our chart, please, Scot. Make sure nothing has been overlooked. Make sure, Scot. We depend on you.'

" 'I have Jennifer,' he said. 'Everything in your chart is on schedule and all your meds and tests are as they should be.'

"I thanked him and hung up. La, we need Scot. We can't forget that. We can't do without him," Jennifer presssed on.

"I'm sure he'll check each detail closely himself. Maybe it's good that it happened," I said.

"We must think so. He's all we have, and La, we will have a baby. You and I will make it happen."

"Yes, Jen, we will." My heart ached with love. "We are a team— an unbeatable team. I love us, Jen."

The next morning I looked to see if my baby bird had returned to the air conditioner. It was empty. I left some bread on the sill hoping the mother would come. I wondered where they were. I tried to believe that the mother was still with the baby. I never understood why they didn't sleep together. I wondered if father birds ever took charge of rearing a baby. It was a foolish thought, I know, but I couldn't help thinking it.

Either way, there was family taking care of family. I missed that baby bird and hoped that he was safe and healthy and happy, and that hopefully, soon, I would have my own baby to fill my nursery with life and miracles.

*I*t was January 11, and day eleven on Lupron. I wasn't getting the daily headaches as I had during the other cycles, but I still felt anxious. Little things at work that normally wouldn't have bothered me now set me off—for example, if a customer made a reservation and didn't call to cancel. My inability to get a straight answer from a nurse enraged me more than I knew it should have.

It was hard to know if it was the Lupron making me testy or if it was the combination of starting IVF and having Jen as gestational carrier, worrying about David's upcoming surgery to collect sperm, and having to interview for a new chef because the current one was too slow and wasteful in the kitchen. At any moment I felt as if I was going to have a heart attack.

It was a hectic Monday night at the restaurant. There was an anniversary party in the back room and a bridal shower in the main dining room. I was thinking of Jen all night, but wasn't able to call until closing. Jen was to start the estrogen patches that night. I knew she must have had trouble with those because of her allergy to the adhesive.

"How'd you do?" I asked when she picked up the phone.

"It wasn't easy to find a spot on my big tush not already covered with welts or scratch marks from the preparatory cycle. Scot called me this evening to tell me that in Japan they administer estrogen in pill form because many women there have sensitive skin like me. But, he said the pills are not as effective as the patches. I want to do this the best way. I'll continue with the patches even though I look like a baboon with this red bottom. Very cute." She laughed and I was so glad that she could still find humor in her predicament.

I awoke the next morning with a terrible headache and my back ached. I hadn't slept well. My right arm felt numb. It wasn't pins and needles, it was lack of sensation, and it frightened me. If my blood was not circulating properly and not flowing to my arms, then I surmised there was a problem elsewhere. I was afraid I would have a stroke. These were the symptoms I'd had on Greg's boat. I called the hematologist at Cornell. He said it was nothing. When a doctor says "it's nothing," I don't feel any peace of mind. I think either they don't know or they aren't telling me something. Then I conclude that really they just don't care.

David told me not to worry; he read in one of my books on IVF that the medicines may interfere with circulation in the extremities. Nevertheless, I continued to worry and had no sleep that night. I kept waiting for something to happen.

In the morning I went to Cornell to have the blood tests, urine test, cultures, and sonogram that Scot had requested. I had never met Dr. Perin, who did the tests. He was surprisingly pleasant and didn't make me wait. He told me I would probably start Metrodin that night, to hyperstimulate my ovaries. He would call after studying the tests. After leaving Cornell, I went to see my family physician, Dr. Robbins, to discuss my numbness and anxiety, hoping to get a fuller understanding of my overall condition. So much attention had been given to reproduction that I was afraid another—perhaps a life-threatening condition—was being overlooked. He said that he agreed that the Lovenox was a great prophylactic medication. He suggested that if I continued to have the anxiety when I finished with all the medicines for the cycle, I might try Xanax to help me relax and help me realize that the anxiety attacks were simply that and not a symptom of anything greater.

Later, I told David of Dr. Robbins's evaluation, thinking he would share in my relief. Instead, his reaction was, "He's not a psychiatrist. Before you think of Xanax, speak to a specialist."

Now I felt rotten, thinking that David was critical of me for the emotional state I was in.

I found comfort discussing this with Jennifer, because she tends to react the same way I do. We were both filled with medicines and hormones that seemed to do whatever they wanted with our emotions. Jennifer got angry when a nurse "forgot" or when doctors didn't return calls, and this reaction seemed normal to me. David brushed such things off saying, "Relax, don't let it bother you." He just doesn't see things as Jen and I do.

That night I was reading my Resolve newsletter. Lately, I anxiously waited to receive it, to learn of the lastest happenings in the world of infertility. It mentioned that Metrodin could be administered through a needle two sizes smaller than the ones I had been instructed to use.

I called Hanna, my next-door neighbor, to ask which needles she used.

"Meet me at the door in three minutes," she said.

I opened the door to find Hanna with a huge, light blue Tiffany shopping bag. She reached inside and looked through an assortment of syringes, needles, alcohol pads, and vials of medication.

"I used these," she said, handing me a green packet of needles.

"These do look a little better," I said. "Could you spare a couple?"

"Take it all," Hanna told me. "I'm done with this stuff, thank goodness. I hope it brings you the luck we have had."

On Thursday, day eighteen of our cycle, I had my first big shot of Metrodin to hyperstimulate my ovaries and cause them to release multiple eggs. Fortunately, when I was at Cornell, I asked Kathy if I could possibly get a prescription for a thinner needle than the one they gave me. She said, "Sure, why not?" I wondered why they hadn't prescribed them initially, as they make the shots considerably less frightening and less painful.

In the evening, David gave me the injection after a lot of talk, anxiety, and procrastinating on my part. He gave it to me in my right hip while I leaned over the bathroom sink to take the weight off my right leg. It hurt, but not as much as I had worked myself up into believing it would. The thinner needle made the difference; just the sight of it was less menacing than the other.

The next afternoon, I met Hanna for tea. Her tummy had grown full and round. She had just installed a washer/dryer in her apartment, getting ready for the twins. Seeing her happy, looking forward to the birth, was balm to my emotional state. It had been a year since I had slipped on ice at Dr. Owins's office going for the pregnancy test after the Fairfax cycle. That winter of '96 had been harsh. Everything was different this year, a different climate completely.

A week before the egg retrieval, which was scheduled the same day as David's surgery, my mother invited us for dinner. I didn't like cooking when I was taking drugs. Preparing food took my appetite away, and going out to a restaurant seemed like work to me. Being in the business myself, I watched for too many details and couldn't relax. It was pleasant being with my mother and her boyfriend, Joe. They had a solid relationship, were physically at ease together, and their camaraderie was obvious. Their love affair had everything—laughter, commitment, and respect. It gave me joy to see them together.

David and Joe had many mutual friends and acquaintances in the advertising business and had in fact worked together at the same agency for a while. After David got over the shock of becoming Joe's "son-in-law," it became a joke between us. "Who would have thought?" we'd say. David and Joe laughed together and my mother and I guessed they might even have dated the same women years ago. We had fun times, the four of us.

During coffee and apricot pie, David brought up my nervousness about the numbness I'd experienced in my arm, and my sleeping difficulties. He candidly said I should see a psychotherapist. He believes in therapy as one way to get a person through their problems. I argued that for me the problem was less daunting than the inability to act on it one way or the other. "We still have an infertility problem, David, but we are doing something about it. Something other than talk," I said with evident hostility. The conversation brought out the differences between my view of life and David's, and frankly, that scared me.

Joe and my mother did not interfere, though I knew their way of thinking. My mother is one to analyze a predicament, find a remedy she can handle, and act on it. Joe would be in accord with David. He believes that having a psychologist you can trust is a real blessing. David and I would hopefully arrive at our goals in our own ways. He with a map, and me—any way it took.

Everything seemed topsy-turvy, up in the air. As supportive as David was being, I was aware of a distance between us. Maybe it was from the drugs. I could be secure and happy one moment and plunge into depression a second later. I wished David would hold and hug me more often. I needed a sense of strength and togetherness. I wanted to believe we were unified and that nothing could separate us, but I couldn't say these things to him. I found it hard to say anything about the way I felt or how I thought we should go about things; he would turn it around and say that I was trying to control him and that he felt as if nothing he did was right.

I asked him to prepare the Metrodin shot. He started unwrapping the syringes. Not knowing there was a starter flap to pull, he began ripping the package open. All I did was tell him, "Pull the tab and it will open easily," but he became very angry, slammed it down, and left the room. Anything I said he took personally.

One night the Lovenox shot wouldn't go in because of the toughening and bruising of my skin from all the previous injections. I was feeling overwhelmed and started to cry. I hated what all this was doing to David and me. I wished it wasn't so difficult, that it could bond us more. I was afraid that the strain of this long ordeal might break us up.

My belly was starting to get that bloated feeling. It was filled with eggs.

*O*n Tuesday, day twenty-one, the radiologist, Dr. Klein, said he saw three or four follicles; they were still small and this was a good indication that more eggs might develop. "Please, please," I breathed, "let more appear." I had had fourteen to eighteen follicles with my first cycle. Tomorrow, he told me, he would have a better sense of the earliest day to expect retrieval.

On Wednesday morning David and I went to Cornell. The waiting room for radiology was exceptionally busy. We waited an hour until Dr. Klein was able to do my sonogram. He said he saw little change from the previous day—four follicles were still small. Again he said, "We'll know better tomorrow; perhaps the estrogen levels will increase and there will be evidence of more eggs." I guess it bears repeating that the entire cycle depended on my being able to create healthy eggs to harvest and fertilize.

I came home feeling disheartened. We had anticipated seeing more follicles than the day before. To rid myself of rising doubts—a repeat of the pessimism I felt before my retrieval at the Fairfax Clinic—I agreed to take a walk in Central Park with Allison, my friend who had undergone IVF, had a child, and was now pregnant with her second. She was full of encouragement, telling me she felt no different during this "natural" pregnancy than she had during her previous IVF pregnancy. She and her husband were moving from New York City to a house in Connecticut, where she would have more room to raise her kids.

"If Jennifer has a multiple birth, David and I will have to move also," I said. I had been unable to think of anything but prescriptions, injections, eggs and sperms, and cell growth for so long that it felt strange to recognize that other issues existed in my life and other people had moved on after they finished IVF and had had a child. My world had shrunk and my thoughts orbited obsessively around infertility. But at least now I was thinking of the baby as a reality, not *if* there *would be* a baby. It was a positive thought.

During our walk, I felt bloated and heavy and too tired to continue fighting the cold wind. I came home to lie down. David called from the office. He was nervous, more than he'd been before. A week before the retrieval, we were both weary but tried desperately to keep our spirits up.

"Liza," he said, his voice full of emotion, "if this doesn't work, we must know, without doubt, that we did the best we possibly could do."

I answered in a stouthearted voice he wasn't used to. "At this moment, I am holding on with desperation to an optimistic view. I practiced my mind trick while walking home from the park. We have three things to be happy about. There are three eggs for certain inside of me and probably a fourth." I think my words made David feel better. When we hung up, I called Jennifer.

"La, in the past you had many more eggs, but were unsuccessful. All we need is one healthy, strong beautiful egg. If you have any more bad thoughts, I'm going to punch you on the right thigh when I see you this weekend."

I laughed, thinking of the still-sore injection site.

"Just know that my mother is here and is going to make this happen," Jennifer said with conviction.

I hung up, amazed at Jennifer's faith. It boosted my spirits. I picked myself up and went to the restaurant to greet my customers for dinner.

It was good being at the restaurant. David came in late and we had dinner at a corner table. It was much better being in the world of busy people than sitting idle at home, where doubt was thick enough to cut with a knife. I was a person of action and the best action I could take was to keep my mind focused on one true thought—we wanted a baby and we would have one. With that in mind, I was able to comfort my husband, assuring him we would get through this. I had turned what would have been another long day of anxious waiting into a day of faith. I slept well that night.

The following day I was confident. I stood tall and I felt empowered. I went to the hospital to have my daily sonogram and my blood and estrogen checks. My estrogen level was up to six hundred, which was great. From there I went to my mother's for breakfast. She was putting loose photos into the family album. We reminisced about the times we had in Spain—how she and I sold bandannas, a piece of America, at the beach restaurant in exchange for lunch. I inserted a photo of me with different-colored bandannas on my hair, neck, and wrist. I realized again that I had not made a mistake in deciding to leave Rafael and have my own children.

Greg met us and we went to the armory to see an exhibit of eighteenth-century paintings; we had a lunch of sandwiches, and orange juice at the small terraced enclosure amid the huge landscapes and pastoral scenes. After the art show, I rested at Mom's apartment and then David joined us with Joe at Greg's restaurant, Bistro Le Steak, for dinner. Greg sat with us while he signed the payroll checks. It was a wonderful day and I was in a good mood. By my own power I had averted that threatening pit of depression.

During the week, as we approached retrieval, I worried about the quality of my eggs, David's surgery, and whether the doctor would be able to collect enough viable sperm. And I worried about Jennifer, and if in reality her commitment to being pregnant was as strong as her dream.

Four days before the retrieval I arrived at Cornell at 9:15 A.M. There wasn't an empty chair in the waiting room. I leaned against the windowsill and thought of Jen's arrival on Sunday, and the fun we'd have just being together; I thought of my birthday the following month. I thought of being with David for the weekend. I knew I was happy. I was healthy, my restaurant was running smoothly. I liked my new chef. We're nearing the end of the cycle, I told myself. Jennifer loves me, Greg loves me, my mother loves me. They love me because I'm myself. That was more than three things.

I wondered if the other women in the waiting room felt as lucky and loved as I did. These women with somber expressions perusing magazines, they no longer angered me. I wasn't jealous of those women with pregnant bellies and I felt true kinship with the other women who like me were trying desperately to have a child. I was the luckiest of women. Oh, how different my life was this year, knowing I would have a baby, I put my hand on my stomach, felt the warmth of my body through my clothes, and envisioned the four egg-filled follicles that Dr. Klein had seen on my last sonogram. Hopefully they weren't too crowded in there, sharing nutrients. They were growing, and getting stronger. I had been taking care of myself to make them as good as they could be. I drank two quarts of water a day, and ate plenty of fruit and vegetables, three meals a day, and I had been sleeping at night.

"Eggs are growing," Dr. Klein reported with a smile sometime later. "It looks good." I walked out feeling that positive things were happening.

Mom was waiting for me and had made a salad for lunch. She asked me to choose one of her sculptures to put on my porch over-looking the garden at the house. It was an easy decision. I selected a life-size hawk swooping down with outstretched wings. It fit the image I carried of my baby bird—grown now, living fiercely and free.

Sunday morning I was up at dawn with one thought: Jennifer is coming today. I felt like I had when we were little girls in the big house on Long Island. I couldn't believe she would actually be here, and in a few days would be flying back to Chicago with our embryos inside her body. That day of the transfer would, in a sense, be my baby's birthday. It would be the day of his physical conception, but his essence—that had been alive and strong for two and a half years. Oh, my baby, I thought, soon your heart will begin to beat.

Stephen was unable to accompany Jennifer because he had a business conference, but he would be home in the evening with Kodie and Austin. This didn't worry Jennifer. She told me: "Lollipop, we're doing this together. You'll be with me." She would go from La Guardia Airport to Queens to visit her father and then arrive at our apartment in time for dinner.

It seemed that Jen and I had been doing this cycle forever, but this was the very last stage and the timing was more crucial than ever. Although it was Sunday, I went to the clinic to see Dr. Klein for my sonogram. He saw seven follicles, some very large—seven to eighteen millimeters, others from twelve to thirteen millimeters—and said there was a greater than 50 percent chance that I would be taking the HCG (human chorionic gonadotropin shot) that night. The HCG causes the eggs to be released from the follicles and must be administered thirty-six hours before retrieval to ensure the viability of the eggs. Therefore, David's sperm aspiration and the retrieval of my eggs would be done simultaneously on Tuesday. The eggs would be immediately fertilized by ICSI and on Friday the embryos would be transferred into Jennifer's lush uterus.

After leaving my mother, I began preparing the apartment for Jennifer's arrival. First I visited the florist. Jennifer liked spring blossoms, irises and pink roses loosely arranged in tall crystal vases. I had two bouquets for the guest room—the room that would soon be my baby's nursery. I bought a dramatic, twisting orchid plant that grew almost magically from a piece of bark, for the dining-table centerpiece. And in the bathroom, on the windowsill behind the tub, I put a red tulip plant so she could relax in bubble bath and look out at the cityscape beyond. I had tiger lilies for the cocktail table in the living room. A bottle of sparkling apple cider, a substitute for champagne, was chilling in an ice bucket. I hoped the more titillating bubbly would not be missed. Pavarotti's voice rang out on the stereo and there were baskets of fruit on the kitchen counter and on the dining-room buffet. I was having so much fun. I planned to order dinner from Sambuca; that way Jennifer would not be tempted to help in the kitchen, and I was so bloated it was uncomfortable to stand up very long much less cook.

The apartment looked welcoming. Everything was in order—the bed turned down, the down quilt fluffy at the bottom. I unwrapped a big bottle of Opium perfume, Jennifer's scent, and placed it in front of the mirror on the bureau. It is sweet and spicy like the medley of flowers, fruits, and potpourri cachets I had set about. Jennifer's primary sense was smell. It set her mood. It was her point of reference when she evaluated the atmosphere of a room. Her acutely sensitive nose would inhale the full bouquet of my love.

As the grandfather clock in the foyer chimed seven o'clock, I knew that Jennifer would arrive any minute. My heart was pounding. When I saw her at the door, I had a sensation I'd never before experienced. I felt as if I was outside my body watching the two of us, two women creating a miracle.

David came home while we were still standing in the hallway gazing at each other. Jen was astonished at my puffy stomach and I held her coat while she mooned me with her red-splotched butt. We were laughing and wiping our tears, making loud sniffing sounds. David put Jen's suitcase in the guest room. They both raved about the apartment and David cracked a joke, saying he wished I made half the fuss over him. We sat in the living room and enjoyed the cider by the candlelight until dinner was delivered.

Scot called while we were twirling pasta on our forks. He said he had received the report from Dr. Klein: the eggs were in position and I could take the HCG shot that night.

At exactly nine-thirty David gave me the injection while Jennifer held my hand. Then we three piled in my bed and watched television. I must have fallen asleep. I didn't hear Jennifer tiptoe out to her room.

I was dreaming of my beautiful eggs and that very soon my baby would be conceived.

*W*e were counting down the hours before egg retrieval.

Jen and I spent the morning at the Cornell Clinic. We each had blood tests and sonograms. She had what they called a trial transfer; it was really an exam; they fitted the catheter they would use to transfer the embryos through her cervix into the uterus to rule out the presence of any obstruction. Dr. Klein saw eight follicles and Jennifer's lining and "sounding" (another test for density) indicated her uterus was perfectly prepared to accept the embryos.

At noon we got to my mother's. Jennifer was so excited, she seemed to prance into the living room. Grandma Reese, who was also there, kept touching Jennifer and me. To her mind, what we were doing was nothing short of witchcraft. We spent a "ladies' afternoon." Jennifer washed and styled Grandma's light auburn hair into a fluffy feather cut and put a natural beige foundation on her cheeks. She replaced the iridescent blue that had been smeared on her eyelids with a smoky shadow. I sat on the white wicker four-poster bed watching the transformation.

"Aunt Suzy, when are you going to repaint the walls in this bedroom? They're Pepto-Bismol pink," Jennifer blurted at one point. "They're shocking."

"Yes, but they make me look pretty when I wake up in the morning."

"The only natural beauty here is you, Grandma. Nothing can make up for a marvelous bone structure," I said.

Grandma was seated in front of the oval mirror at my mother's vanity table. "I wish you had known my mother," she said, peering at her transformed image. "She was an adorable woman and such fun. She died when I was ten years old." She looked up at Jennifer. "Where's your mother, darling? She called me this morning."

Jennifer shot me a baffled look. "That was me, Grams."

"Oh, yes, of course. Sometimes your grandmother is a goose." She blinked her eyes as Jen brushed brown mascara onto her lashes.

"Okay, everyone. What do you think?" Jen stepped back to get the full picture. "A little blush and you're done."

Grandma looked pleased. "Laurie, you've made me beautiful." Hearing the error, Jennifer's face was filled with compassion.

"Grandma," I said, deliberately changing the subject, "I'm going to the kitchen, would you like a cup of tea?"

"No, dear. Tell Ruby I'm ready to leave now. I want the girls at the home to see my face." She rose unsteadily to her feet.

"I called the car service. They'll be here in ten minutes," I said, trying to keep her calm and seated while she waited for the cab.

She looked carefully at her watch. "I'm ready, I want to go now. Ruby, dear, bring my coat. We can't keep them waiting."

The companion took Grandma's arm and led her into the hallway.

"Is she always so confused?" Jen asked, her face still tight.

"No, Jen," my mother said, "she's mixed up today. Your story unsettled her, partly because she doesn't pay attention and partly because she doesn't want to understand. Grandma hasn't changed. She's an actress and chooses to live out the dramas in her own mind."

"Do you visit her often?" Jen asked.

"Every week."

"I'm glad."

We went down in the elevator with Grandma and Ruby and

helped them into the car, then we crossed the street for a manicure. Jennifer had a French manicure on her stilettolike nails. The white-polished tips made them appear even longer. I had "Ballet Slipper" painted on mine, the same demure pink I'd worn for my wedding.

At home I washed my hair and blew it straight, which gave me a more composed appearance than my usual unruly curls. Jennifer said she would get up early in the morning to blow-dry her hair, which was always perfectly styled.

To both Jen and me, our appearance was especially important that day. We were being judged from the inside where we had no control, but at least we could exercise some control over what people saw on the outside. Jennifer and I agreed—if you look the best, you are the best.

We were all preparing ourselves in our own way for the next day's retrieval and David's surgery, which would happen simultaneously. David was reading the *Times* and doing the crossword puzzle. Jennifer was making cookies to have with tea before we went to sleep. When she brought the tray to the bed, we sat together talking of what would come tomorrow during the next phase of our journey.

Jennifer was up at 5:30 A.M. to be first in the shower, then it was my turn, and then David's. By eight we were at the hospital, manicured, newly coiffed, scrubbed, and polished from head to toe.

We went to the admitting room, which was painted a soft peach color, making the place less austere and impersonal than I'd expected. The receptionist greeted us—and by our correct names! I donned the paper pajamas I was given, and the three of us sat down on peach-colored armchairs to wait.

"Mrs. Freilicher." A nurse came through the swinging door behind the receptionist's desk. "We're ready, you can come with me, please." It was 8:45 A.M.

Jen and David hugged me and watched me walk down the hall to the retrieval room. I marched into the operating room with my back straight and my head up. If ever I needed to use all my powers of positive thinking, it was now. Those eggs were my creation—mine alone, my magnificent contribution to the conception of our child or children, the most important contribution of my life. Think three, I told myself: Liza, David, baby.

The OR nurse introduced herself. "I'm Diane, Liza, and this is the laboratory staff." She took my chart. "Are you still taking Lovenox and one aspirin a day?"

"Yes," I replied, beginning to perspire as she helped me onto the table. She covered me with a sheet and told me to remove my underwear and robe.

"Lie down, please, Liza."

Immediately one of the technicians prepped my arm and started an IV. One quick pinch. It didn't hurt.

Diane patted my shoulder. "You'll be fine. From your chart I see you have promising eggs. Try to relax." She took my hand; that is the last I remember until I awoke in the recovery room. I was still hooked up to the IV and my stomach felt crampy, otherwise I didn't feel sick. A strange nurse removed the IV and helped me sit up. When the room stopped spinning I got into a wheelchair and was pushed to the recovery lounge.

"How many eggs did the doctor get?" I asked.

"I'm sorry. You'll have to ask your doctor."

I lay in the reclining chair and drank ginger ale and ate Ritz crackers—to minimize my nausea. I wasn't apprehensive. They got good eggs, I told myself, stay calm. I went into the bathroom; there was no blood. When I came out Jen and David were there, smiling.

"Nine eggs," David announced, and embraced me. I rested my head on his shoulder.

"We did well," I murmured as relief washed over me.

Jen helped me get dressed. "Nine beauties. Dr. Klein met us as they were pushing you into the recovery room."

"Nine." David held me and wiped my tears—tears of joy. "Nine eggs."

We went back to the waiting room and listened for David's name to be called for his procedure. He wasn't worried. We held hands. We had nine eggs. We sat, the three of us, not saying a word, holding hands . . . united.

Soon an orderly came to get David. He said we could accompany him only as far as the elevator. When the door slid closed, Jen and I returned to the waiting room. It would be a few hours.

Dr. Seagal, David's urologist, came in and sat down to talk to us. "David did well. We have several specimens of healthy sperm. We have enough to freeze."

That was good news. If we wanted to fertilize eggs in the future, David would not have to endure another invasive surgery.

"Come. You can see him now."

We followed Dr. Seagal to the recovery room, where we found David awake, smiling weakly, and overjoyed at the success of the procedure. He said he had been awake for most of the surgery, talking to Dr. Seagal, asking questions. He had little pain.

David drank and ate some crackers, had his IV removed, and went to the bathroom. He was ready to go.

I helped him dress and we were out of there, in a cab, and on our way home.

Back in our apartment, David and I put on cozy clothes. Jen made dinner. She wouldn't let me help. We had tuna sandwiches and potato chips and matzoh-ball soup that Jennifer's father had left for us with the doorman. It was a simple meal, but I don't remember anything ever tasting so delicious. We turned off the phone and got in bed and took a long nap. David felt stronger after the rest. I still had cramps and a feeling of pressure in my stomach, but after two Tylenol, it went away. We sat together in our big bed making phone calls—I to the restaurant and Jennifer to Chicago. She looked worried. Kodie had been nipped on the cheek by her friend's dog, and Christine had taken her to the doctor.

The wound was cleaned and probably wouldn't leave a scar, but Kodie had been badly shaken. Jennifer consoled her with gentle words. It was a minor incident, but Jennifer's inability to be with her child, who only wanted to feel the safety of her mother's arms about her, seemed a big sacrifice to me. Being a mother was more than having a baby.

Greg came up to visit. He brought a chocolate mousse cake from Bonte, his favorite French bakery, and dished it out among us.

"We are all so lucky to have each other," he said. "I hope Stuart and Sophia grow up feeling as close to Kodie and Austin as we feel to each other."

"Mommy and Aunt Laurie had no cousins. They only had each other," I said.

"We're creating a new generation," Jennifer said. "I imagine a long line of our children, shoulder to shoulder, one next to the other, as they go through life."

"Stuart asks me all the time: when will Aunt La give me a cousin so I can teach him the computer?" Greg said.

We devoured more than half the cake. Before Greg left he brought the dishes into the kitchen. I was looking through the day's mail when Jen announced that it was time for her progesterone shot.

"David, will you give it to me?"

I was proud that she asked my husband—and wasn't surprised that she had. It showed the easy camaraderie that had been established between us. Liza and Jennifer, David and Stephen, what one couldn't do, the other could. There were no barriers between us.

Jen saw David's face flush. "You've seen one rump, you've seen 'em all. Will you do it? I need a man's quickness and strength. Liza says you're great."

The three of us went into the bathroom, where she had the syringe prepared. She used my trick of putting the filled syringe under her armpit so the oil-based medicine would become warm and flow more easily. She bent over the sink as I had. On her butt was a random design of red welts. David found an area of virgin skin on her hip.

"Okay, Jen, are you ready? I don't want to hurt you."

"I'm ready. Go ahead."

I watched him pinch her flesh and inject the needle. "How are you able to sit down?" I asked, swabbing the spot with alcohol.

"Very gently," she replied, grimacing.

We were up early Wednesday morning and by nine o'clock were dressed, had eaten breakfast, and were sitting looking at the telephone, waiting for it to ring. Cornell would be calling us sometime that morning with the fertilization results. As time passed and it approached noon, we were jumping at the slightest sound.

Kathy called from Scot's office a few minutes past noon. "As you know, you had nine eggs. One was immature and didn't make it. Of the nine, five fertilized. That's very good. Generally, you lose half the eggs before you get fertilized ones." She said she wouldn't have any more information about the embryos until Friday.

I closed my eyes and sent a silent message. "Please, my little embryos, be strong and grow; know you have a warm, healthy uterus to live in until you come to live with your parents, who can't wait to hold you and love you and offer you a beautiful life. We are waiting for you. We are thinking of you growing and maturing— being healthy and anxious for your new home."

After having a lunch of lox and bagels, Jen and I went to Cornell for Jennifer's blood test, to check her progesterone and estrogen levels. The nurses congratulated us on our fertilization results. Jennifer spent the afternoon with her father and I stayed home to relax with David. It was a peaceful day. We went to Sambuca for dinner and we were in bed and asleep early.

Thursday, January 30, 1997, was the day before transfer. We had no doctors' appointments or commitments. Jen and I went to the bank and to the Betsy Johnson Boutique to chose a gift for Christine, then on to the Disney Store to find gifts for Kodie, Austin, and Sophia. We bought a video game for Stuart, then we went to Bergdorf Goodman. We walked around the store, browsing randomly. Jen bought me a pair of silver-flower shaped earrings and a gift for Hilary. It felt like a holiday.

It astonishes me how rapidly mundane thoughts and chores come rushing back to fill your life when the most difficult ones have been accomplished.

"Jen," I said, "I want you to pick something out for yourself, otherwise I'll get something you might not like. It has to be special." I didn't know what to do for her. There was no way to repay her or show my gratitude. I hugged her and began to cry, right there in the jewelry department of Bergdorf Goodman.

"Lollipop, I know how you feel. You don't have to buy me anything."

"I want you to have something that you will love and that will always let you know how much I love you."

Two salesladies were listening to us. One asked, "Can I help you? Is something the matter?"

"The matter?" I laughed. "No, everything is marvelous, wonderful. That's why we're here, for a gift to mark this day."

We told them that the following day Jennifer would become the carrier of my biological embryos. The lady who had first spoken to us began to cry; the other showed us the goose bumps our words had caused to appear on her arm, and said it was the most remarkable story she had heard in the fifteen years she'd been at the store.

Jennifer chose a Robert Lee Morris necklace with matching earrings. The necklace was a creation of three loosely hinged free-form gold pieces that rippled downward.

"Jen, they look like wavelets that kiss the shore. See how they move?" I picked up the pieces from the velvet tray.

"Remember how we used to go to the beach with our mothers when we were little?"

"We used to walk and walk holding hands."

"And Aunt Suzy would tell us stories about mermaids who lived in the ocean and granted wishes for each pure white pebble that was thrown back to them into the waves."

"We had pails of pebbles. You must have wished for greatness, Jen."

"No, I wished I didn't have to go to school. I was always afraid to leave Mommy. I wished to be as brave as you were, La." She held the necklace up so the light glistened on the curves of swaying gold.

"I wasn't brave. I hated school and the clique of kids. I've always been a loner. I wished I was beautiful and looked like a princess, like you."

"We both got our wishes granted. Liza, I don't need a necklace or any tangible memento for these days."

I took the necklace from Jennifer and fastened the clasp behind her neck. It filled the opening at the throat of her blazer. "Yes," I whispered. "Oh, yes."

"It's beautiful," Jen said, and touched the gold. Then she lifted her hair and flirted with the mirror. "Can you imagine if those mermaids knew what we were doing? If they schemed it?"

"Mermaids are fantasy. We are real." I signaled to the saleslady, who had discreetly turned away to give us privacy. "We'll take it."

"La, I'll wear it always," Jen said. "Starting now!" Her eyes glinted and she strutted out of the store, the gold necklace on her neck gleaming as she moved.

My mother and Greg had planned a dinner celebration that evening at Marchi's, a family-run Northern Italian restaurant in a town house in the Kips Bay area of the city. Our family had been customers there for many years. The atmosphere is homey, and because we were regulars the owners gave us a private dining room with flowers and candlelight. In the center of the long table were three platters of Marchi's traditional appetizers of leafy vegetables, melons, cheeses, and salamis. Jennifer and I were there early to have time to freshen our makeup in the ladies' room.

My mother arrived with Erica. My sister looked beautiful: her slim doll-like body, her thick blond hair falling as free as her spirit in her signature black bodysuit and black jeans. It saddened me to think that through the years we always seemed to miss each other. Either I was in school or in Europe; our lives barely touched. She flitted between her own schooling and various jobs with what seemed to me a numbness to passion to which I could not relate. Perhaps that was why we were never really friends.

Greg and Max showed up with Stuart in a gray suit and one of his father's ties. Sophia resembled a Victorian doll in a long red velvet and lace dress.

Stanley came, too. He was alone, which was considerate of him. If he'd brought his wife, Jennifer would have been uncomfortable.

"I'm glad to be included in this family gathering," he said, employing his trademark of noncommittal good cheer.

"You are family," Jennifer replied.

"And always will be," my mother added.

During dinner, Jen sat next to Stanley. From across the table, I watched her body language as they spoke. She was leaning back comfortably in the chair and her hands were still. If she was agitated, she would have been fingering the silverware or the edge of her napkin. I didn't know what they were saying, but if I'd been close enough, I'd have heard Stanley say, "This is so typically you, Jen. It goes along with who you are. Your mother would be proud of you." He didn't ask any questions.

"I'm glad you came. This is an evening of spiritual healing for me. A celebration. It's what Mommy would have wanted and I appreciate hearing you say so."

Erica made an excuse and left early. I sensed she was intimidated by our hurrahs.

Before the cake and the coffee were served, while the table was being cleared and waiters finished rattling dishes, I stood up. Everyone looked at me—I hadn't prepared any words to say; my feelings simply poured forth while I gasped and tried to regain my composure. "I can't express all my love and gratitude to my beautiful Jennifer, and my husband for the miracle that is about to happen. Jen and David, you gave me the strength and faith to believe. You gave the stuff of your own life. And Stephen, thank you for your support. And Mommy, you and Greg and you, my Stuart, who understand the heart better than a grown-up and are wiser than me, opened my eyes to the blessings that surround me. How fortunate that we are here today in a world that has the technology to make our dreams possible. But . . ." And here I sniffed and gulped like a dope. "But the greatest miracle is all of us together. My family." I sat down.

David stood up. "Jen, Liza. The two women I respect most in the world. I love you. I am filled with awe. You have given me a new life that soon I'll be holding in my arms and everyone will look at me and say . . . shut that damn kid up . . ."

We all laughed.

Next, Jennifer stood. She was beaming. She touched the gold at her throat as she spoke. "Thanks, guys, for letting me be part of this birth day. And thank you, Mommy, for giving me the light and teaching me to trust."

My mother raised her hand. She nodded and tried to speak, but after a pause she merely said, "Look in my eyes and read my heart. There are no words for what you will see there for each of you."

A moment earlier, Mother was treated to a glimpse of what will always be the most memorable moment of that evening: David standing with his arms around Jennifer and me.

January 29, 1997

Aunt Suzy doesn't have to tell me, but I see the question in her eyes. Am I mad or jealous that she is here, alive, and my mother—her sister—is not? I am jealous of Liza for having her mother. I wish Aunt Suzy could walk. I wish there was no pain and we were all here. She tries to treat me with a sort of reserved maternity, but sees I reject it. It is because no one can take my mother's place and I can't fool myself or her that it does.

Tomorrow, when I leave the hospital with the embryos in my womb, it will be the start of healing all these ragged edges, and when the baby or babies are born I will have healed the core and Liza will have her family.

*F*riday, January 31, 1997, was the day of the transfer. On this day of days Jennifer and I woke early. We had breakfast with David before he went to work and made plans for him to pick us up at the apartment at eleven A.M. We would park the car at the hospital so Jennifer would be comfortable and have a safe ride home. I didn't put much faith in the New York taxi drivers; the trip would be jolting at best.

At noon we were at the Cornell Clinic. We waited in a dismal corridor with five seats. It wasn't as pleasant as the place where we had waited for the retrieval, but it was outside the same OR that was also the embryologist's laboratory.

The nurse came and gave Jennifer and me our green paper pajamas, which we promptly donned. Soon we were called into the OR and were thrilled to learn that Dr. Klein was the doctor doing the transfers that day.

The nurse smiled and said, "Now just one of you lie down on the table."

I held Jen's hand as she lay down and was draped with a sheet.

Dr. Klein told us, "You have four embryos. Three with eight cells, and one with seven." He looked pleased.

Jen squeezed my hand. This was good news. I had been nervous that the embryos might be of low cell count, as they had been at Fairfax.

He showed us a picture of the embryos on a large television screen. I remember thinking they looked like flowers. "I'll give you a photo of these before you go home. I suggest you transfer all four embryos. It is best we use all our chances."

Jennifer's face tightened, and I knew why.

"We were told generally three embryos are transferred," I said.

"Yes, but with women over thirty-five, I recommend transferring the four. There is a forty-five percent chance of multiple births, most of that number being twins. Often more than one embryo will adhere to the uterus but not make it to term."

I could see from Jennifer's face that she was frightened. We looked at each other. Here was the decision we had tried to prepare for.

We had gone over this issue much earlier with Scot. He told us he would probably implant three embryos if we had that many. I preferred one healthy baby. Jen liked the idea of twins. Triplets had been ruled out. But that was before we started, when everything was speculation and talk. Now we were faced with living embryos. Suddenly the rules had changed.

"Can't we freeze an embryo?" I asked.

"Liza, there's a risk that the embryo will not survive the freezing and it certainly won't maximize your chances to have a baby."

I looked at Jen. Without blinking an eye, she said, "Okay, give 'em all to me."

I held her hand while the four embryos were transferred. She thought she had known what to expect since she had undergone a practice procedure the day before and I had given her detailed accounts of my experiences. Nevertheless, as she and I watched the screen and observed the embryos being gently placed in her uterus, it all seemed new.

Jennifer's face was pink and her eyes wide. She was accepting a gift. And me? I was watching my babies being tucked away to be nurtured and loved until I would hold her/him/them. It was a gift

from heaven, those flowers, those embryos. Each with its own genetic package. Each the sum and substance of an individual. Which
would have the staying power to be born?

The procedure was quick and practically painless.

"I'm pleased with the embryos. Cell division is what it should be.
I wish you all luck," the doctor summed up.

When the transfer was complete, Jennifer and I clasped our hands
over her stomach. The nurse wheeled her to a recovery area and
gave David the photograph of the four embryos now in Jennifer's
uterus. He and I marveled at those tiny blooms.

Jennifer rested for half an hour, then a nurse with a lovely Islands
accent told us we could go.

Jennifer and I got dressed. She put on her high heels and we
walked to meet David, who had gone ahead to get the car. I watched
every step she took, wishing she were wearing sneakers and repri-
manding myself for thinking I could control her. Jennifer would
always wear her high heels.

Jennifer sat in the backseat of the car. I had lain down in the car
on the way home and I was thinking it would be better if she were
to do the same. I wondered if this was a sign of things to come for
the next nine months. Would I bother Jennifer, demanding to know
what she was eating, how many hours she slept, or how long she
had been on her feet or how much of the day she had spent walking?
Would I be as invasive about her personal life as I had been about
her physical life? I didn't want to be a controlling figure. I made a
conscious effort to stop myself before it became an obsession.

At home I helped Jennifer into her nightgown and made some
sandwiches while she watched television on David's and my bed.
We ate at the dining room table. On the embroidered tablecloth, I
set out all the fine crystal and china I had received as wedding
gifts. By eleven o'clock we were tired. Jennifer went to sleep in the
guest room, soon to be a nursery. I tucked her into bed like a little girl.

I woke up at seven and still felt tired. It was dark outside. I went
to wake Jen, but she was already in the bathroom blow-drying her
hair; she had packed and was ready to go to the airport. We had

breakfast at La Guardia and waited until it was time for her to board the plane. I thought it would be a teary departure, but it wasn't. Jennifer wanted to be home.

February 1, 1997

I am flying home to my babies in Chicago in an airplane filled to capacity with everyday people. I am unique and I have a secret. I'm surprised no one has felt shocks from the energy surging through my body. I am a fox.

DAVID AND I DROVE to our house on Long Island. I called Jennifer in the late afternoon figuring she was home resting after her trip. Christine answered to say Jennifer was with Kodie at the doctor. When, at last, she called back, she said it had been a smooth plane ride home, Kodie's cheek was healing well; she had already gone marketing and done the laundry. At that moment, she was in the kitchen preparing dinner, already back in her whirlwind routine. I took a breath and didn't utter a single word of protest.

Chapter
36

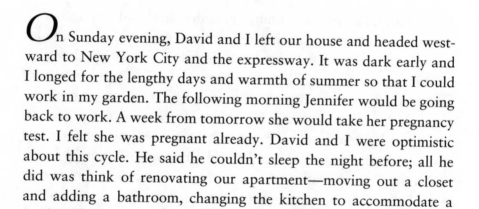

On Sunday evening, David and I left our house and headed west-
ward to New York City and the expressway. It was dark early and
I longed for the lengthy days and warmth of summer so that I could
work in my garden. The following morning Jennifer would be going
back to work. A week from tomorrow she would take her pregnancy
test. I felt she was pregnant already. David and I were optimistic
about this cycle. He said he couldn't sleep the night before; all he
did was think of renovating our apartment—moving out a closet
and adding a bathroom, changing the kitchen to accommodate a
washer/dryer.

"David, have you thought of what we'll do if Jennifer isn't pregnant—if we aren't pregnant?" I asked.

"I guess we would have to adopt. You wouldn't go through all
this again," he answered.

"I wouldn't ask Jennifer, and for me it's a health risk, but now
we have our own sperm frozen; it would be tempting and frustrating
not to be able to use them," I said, though I had no particular plan
in my mind.

"Liza, the way technology is moving, in a few years we might be
able to use my frozen sperm with your egg in another situation. Who
knows what they will come up with?" David was always hopeful.

And I was always impatient. "We don't have time to wait for technology. I'm thirty-six years old already. I'd like to be prepared with a backup plan should it turn out that we're not pregnant. But I don't think we'll get to that. Please, please, I pray, let this be successful. If this doesn't work, we will all be so devastated."

That night, I got my period. I was off the Lovenox injections; Jen was still taking progesterone.

The following Sunday night, Jen called us in New York at eleven P.M. We had just gotten home and David was parking the car. She said she had been nauseous all morning, and had no signs that her period was coming. She was well and energetic, she reported. However, she noticed a difference in her sense of smell. She said it was more acute than usual, as it had been during her last pregnancy. I wondered if it was merely wishful thinking.

Sometimes what we were doing seemed radical and outrageous. If someone had mentioned using a gestational carrier as a solution for infertility problems a few years ago, I would have thought they were talking science fiction. Now it seemed to be just another way of having a baby. I knew more people who were trying to get pregnant through reproductive technology than the way of the proverbial birds and bees; still, it was hard to believe I was one of them. Of my friends and acquaintances I could name ten, all women in my age group. My generation would produce a new community of children. I remember when my parents decided to divorce, my mother was so upset about telling me. I was seventeen years old. I said, "Ma, why are you worried? All my friends' parents are divorced." That was my generation of kids. And now it is children who result from assisted pregnancies—desperately wanted children.

These were strange times, times that naturally led to serious soul-searching. I thought of Carol and Randy and the love they had for their adopted child, Jake. I thought of the lesson I had taught myself at the museum in D.C. as I marveled at the speed and the feats of technology. I remembered the insight of love I had found at the horse ranch and knew that over the past year I had grown emotionally. I thought of Stuart and Greg and how their help had made me open myself up to change. I thought of the great love Jennifer had shown. And of Stephen's love for her. And David, together with me. And I thought about Aunt Laurie and my mother, and I knew I would love our baby whether he had grown inside Jennifer or a stranger.

Jennifer was convinced that she was pregnant. David and I were praying she was right. In twenty-two hours we would know. If the test was negative, would he criticize me? I wondered. Would I criticize him? Our marriage had been under a lot of stress for a long time, and though each of us responded to stress differently, we were both quick to denounce one another. Nevertheless, we loved each other. Knowing this, I also knew that whatever the news, I needed to trust our bond.

I told Jennifer that whatever the outcome of the pregnancy test, David and I knew her intention had truly been to carry our baby. It was the kindest, most generous, and self-sacrificing act I had ever witnessed. Sometimes I wondered who most wanted this dream fulfilled—David and me or Jennifer. I was no longer filled with suffering for every injection Jennifer had to receive. I believed her joy and it filled me. I was more at peace than I had ever been before.

Chapter

37

*T*en days after our embryos were implanted into Jennifer's uterus, she went for her pregnancy test. In New York, the sky was clear and the air brisk.

I was exhilarated, but not nervous, as I had been when I went for my own tests. I didn't relate that past to the present. "I know this is meant to be. I sense it, I see it," I said to David that morning. There was none of the doom and gloom I had experienced before. David, Jen, and I would be pregnant. The three of us.

We planned for her to call us at two-thirty, or the moment she heard.

"La, stay calm. We have nothing to worry about," she had said before going to the doctor.

David was to come home from his meeting by two o'clock and wait for the call with me.

The phone rang at noon, but I didn't want to answer it. Jennifer wasn't due to call until two o'clock, at the earliest. I finished my set of eight push-ups and grabbed the persistent ringer.

Jennifer and Stephen were screaming with joy. "We're pregnant!"

"What?" I couldn't believe it. "Are you sure?" I didn't know what to say. I couldn't cry or holler. I was incredulous. An explosion of emotion surged through me

Jen got David at the office on a conference line. When he heard the news, he began to cry uncontrollably. I didn't hear him say a word.

"David. David, are you there? Can you believe it?"

Finally I heard his little crying voice. "Oh, my God."

"Jen, how did you find out so soon?" I asked.

"All the nurses and Dr. Isola love me so much they found out early and didn't want me to wait."

I must have said "I can't believe it" one hundred times. Jennifer and Stephen said they had always known the test would come out positive.

"I knew it, too," I said, "but oh, I still can't believe it. I knew it, Jen. Oh, God, Jen."

I pulled on a sweatshirt and took a cab across town to Mom's sculpture studio; I wanted to tell her in person. As I dashed up the two flights of stairs in the converted brownstone, I heard the din of an air compressor over the steady *tap-tap-tap* of hammer meeting chisel. My mother was seated in front of a large piece of marble in a cloud of white stone dust. She was so absorbed in her carving that she hadn't seen me come dashing through the open room.

"Mom."

In one moment, she dropped her tools, ripped off her goggles and face mask, and gripped the arms of her chair expectantly.

"Jen's pregnant."

Her face flushed. She threw her arms around me and cried. She couldn't hold me close enough. Both of us cried against the rhythmic background tapping of her fellow artists, who were being polite and not stopping to pry. We cried and laughed and she hollered out loud, "We're having a baby!" That was when the hammering finally stopped. She hollered out the announcement again and the compressor stopped as well. A group of welders suddenly came stomping in the front room. All her friends, who had been kept abreast of our progress, congratulated me, then took up their tools and the sounds of creation continued.

"Did you tell your father? Call him. Let's call him." Mom dug in her satchel for her cellular phone. "Again, thank goodness for technology." She laughed. "You're covered with dust."

"Who cares? It's beautiful." I spun around.

"La, I'm so happy. Look at you. Look in the mirror over there. You are so beautiful. I never saw anything so beautiful." She hugged me again and wiped her wet eyes, leaving a white streak across her face.

"Can we call Jen? First let's call Jennifer."

I dialed Jennifer's office number and gave the phone to Mom.

"Jen, congratulations. Oh, Jennifer, I don't know what to say. I'm crying. I'm happy for all of us. I love you. How do you feel?"

"Aunt Suzy," Jen whispered, "I'm perfect, but I can't talk at work. No one knows. I'll call you tonight."

"Stephen is happy? You'll tell Kodie? Oh, Jen. I'll call you at home later."

We called my father at his office. After two disconnects and being put on hold by three people at the restaurant, we were able to tell him the news. He sounded excited. The conversation was brief and pleasant at the time, but in retrospect, I realize that I was disappointed by my father's reaction because I really had no idea how he truly felt, if he experienced the enormity of Jennifer being pregnant with our baby, if he understood what a baby of our own meant to David and me, if he comprehended the glorious miracle. He had never shared his problems with me. I have never known what my father felt inside; he only allowed me to know the obvious.

Then we called Greg. "Wow!" he cried, and then I heard him sniffeling.

We called Joe at his office. "I'm a grandpa, again?" he asked, laughing.

My aunt Ilene wanted to know how we were planning to decorate the baby's room, and Grandma Reese was confused, yet understanding the high pitch of excitement in my voice, said she was "thrilled."

Both David and I left work early; we wanted to be together. When we met at home, we held each other tightly, crying and laughing. There was so much excitement in the air.

The phone rang again. This time it was Scot.

"Congratulations, Liza. You're pregnant." He sounded victorious.

"Congratulations to you, too. We told you you'd have a positive statistic for the clinic."

He chuckled. "I spoke to Jen. She'll be going to Dr. Isola in four weeks, about the third of March, for a sonogram. You'll learn then if there is more than one baby and possibly hear a heartbeat."

I gasped. "Thank you, Scot. We couldn't have done it without you."

David and I decided to go out, although neither of us were hungry. We wanted to be alone, to be away from the telephone, to fantasize, plan, and rejoice.

We went to Petrossian, an elegant and well-known Russian restaurant. We wanted to dine someplace special and luxurious. We walked to the restaurant holding hands tightly.

We entered the beautiful building on Seventh Avenue near Central Park and requested an intimate table. Both of us beamed as we thought of our incredible news and exciting secret.

David ordered Perrier and caviar. We toasted to our baby, to Jennifer, to love, to life.

As the night went on, our giddiness subsided. We were reminded of the long road ahead and the many hurdles to overcome. So many "ifs."

However, for this brief moment we were free, triumphant, and delirious about our miracle baby.

February 10, Monday

I knew it. We're pregnant. That proves everything I saw and understood from my hypnotic encounter with Mommy is true. Everything. She is alive inside me and I feel joy.

Chapter
38

February 24, Monday

I have been depressed for two days. Perhaps it was an inevitable letdown after all the excitement. It could be hormonal. Scot said I must stay on the estrogen patches through my third month of pregnancy. He suggested using Benadryl cream on the rashes. The damn things won't stick on the area if I put cream on my skin. He told me I could go on estrogen pills if the patches don't stick, but that the pills are not as effective as the patches. But the patches aren't effective if they don't stick! I dread taking a shower because the water stings the irritation and I hate covering myself out of fear that Dakota will see my inflamed skin. I'll continue the patches and forget the cream.

This afternoon at work I began to feel hot and cold flushes and had a pounding headache. Stephen picked me up at the office and took me home, something I have never done. I was sick to my stomach twice and had a 103-degree temperature. The vomiting frightened me. I called Dr. Isola.

"It doesn't mean you're miscarrying, Jennifer. It sounds like

flu. Drink as much water as you can. I don't want you to get dehydrated."

Her reassurance made me feel better. I'm very tired and going to sleep now. Stephen came in and told me Liza has been calling all afternoon since Ellen told her I left work. She must be in a panic. I'll call her, then I'll go to sleep.

In early March, David and I flew to Chicago to be there for Jen's sonogram. She said she was over the flu that had been a fright for all of us. I brought a package of "Sculpi" for Dakota to mold into farm animals, and some Legos for Austin to build a fort. For Jen I found a large artfully illustrated international cookbook, though she told me she was watching her weight and recently had had no interest in cooking.

We arrived at the house a few minutes after Jen got home from work. Christine had prepared dinner. Jen looked radiant—I think because we were so glad to see each other.

"Jen, do you feel different than you did with Kodie or Austin?" I asked her. "Do you feel like twins, or . . ." I hesitated to say "triplets."

"I feel the same. I think if it were multiple pregnancy, I would be bigger. I'm not bigger . . . yet." She showed me her waistline. "And I feel wonderful, except, when I get home from work, I'm really tired."

After dinner I gave Austin his bath and helped Kodie with her reading homework so Jennifer could go to sleep earlier. I was getting practice being a mom.

The next day we saw our baby for the first time. Jennifer, Stephen, David and I watched the screen as the baby appeared. We saw the fetus, the heart beating, so tiny and perfect. Dr. Isola moved the wand over Jennifer's stomach. There was one baby—one fetus. We were all a bit surprised, but it was a good surprise. Dr. Isola searched the screen, looking to see if there was any debris from other embryos or if there was an ectopic (tubal) pregnancy. Neither Jen nor I had ever been aware of this possibility. No one had mentioned it. But it turned out that everything was clean and clear. The fetus was the appropriate size for its age and the embryonic sac showed the correct proportions. Dr. Isola said there was a 95 percent chance that Jennifer would carry a healthy baby to term. Of course we'd do the amnio test in fifteen to sixteen weeks to rule out any congenital problems. David and I had already undergone rigorous genetic screening to eliminate a number of conditions that were genetically linked. We were hopeful.

Before leaving the office, I gave Dr. Isola and her staff a box of chocolates to show our appreciation for the kindness and understanding they'd shown to Jennifer and to all of us as a team. I felt they cared and were honored to be part of such a bold and loving endeavor. Their thoughtfulness made a difference; it was what I had sorely missed during my IVF cycle.

David and I flew to Florida from Chicago to spend the weekend with his parents. I was resting back in the airplane seat, feeling close to my baby. It was hard to leave Jennifer and "him." Now that I had I seen him, he was my only reality. I had put my hand on Jennifer's stomach, over his beating heart, willing him life and independent power. Wonder of wonders.

In her second month of pregnancy, Jennifer began to feel very tired and told me with formidable resolve that it was only because she was working, which she hadn't done during her previous pregnancies. She had her second sonogram on March 13 and reported, "The baby is twice the size as when we saw him on the first sonogram. I say he, but the sex isn't clear yet. We'll know for sure with the amnio test. The doctor said according to his size, we are eight weeks and six days pregnant. Tomorrow starts our third month. This is going fast."

I sent Jennifer two more vials of progesterone, which I hoped would be her last medications, and a professional hair dryer to cut down on her styling time. I bought her an outfit at a maternity store, The Pea in the Pod. It was fun to go in, browse through the racks, and pretend I was looking for myself. I sent her a black jacket, which I tried on, putting a pillow inside, and black trousers to match. She called to thank me and said her father had come to visit and had commented on how pregnant she looked. I sent her a Polaroid camera so she could take pictures for David and me. I did not consider these items gifts and I don't believe that Jennifer received them that way. Rather, giving her these things that would make the pregnancy easier represented my involvement in it, and I was coming to think of it as my own.

April 1, 1997

It will soon be obvious that I am pregnant. We are in the eleventh week, and I am no longer able to wear my business clothes. My slacks don't close at the waist and my blouses won't button over my breasts, which are now enormous. But before I put on maternity clothes and before anyone knows or suspects my pregnancy, I want to tell Dakota so she will understand why this baby did not belong to us. I was worried she would not grasp how unique and special this was and that the decision was difficult because it affected her life, Austin's, and Stephen's as well as mine.

I told Kodie and Austin together on Saturday morning as we cuddled in my bed and Stephen sat on the chair beside us. I chose to tell them in the morning so they would have the day to think about it. I didn't want them to go to bed with unanswered questions. I explained in words a six-year-old would understand without arousing any new fears. I wanted them to recognize the importance of family and children and how we as a family, working together, could give what we have to Aunt La and Uncle David.

Kodie listened quietly. She sat up and pushed her hair from her face and looked at me as I spoke.

"Aunt La's tummy is not strong enough to hold a baby, so the doctor put their baby, when it was tiny, smaller than a pea, in my tummy. It will grow and become your cousin."

Austin smiled, "Can we see your tummy, Mommy? I want to see the baby."

"He's still too small to see. But soon you will see me get

rounder." I showed them my stomach. Austin patted it and jumped off the bed to go downstairs and tell Baci [the family dog].

Dakota was wise. She wanted to know how I could have a baby that wasn't part of me. "Austin and I are part of you, aren't we?" she asked.

I told her, "The doctors made it possible. They give me medicine and then put the baby inside of me. Daddy gives me the medicine by injection every night."

"I hate shots. They hurt you, don't they, Mommy?"

"Yes, for a moment. You know. But the happiness we'll know when Liza and David have their baby makes it all worthwhile."

"Like I feel when I straighten my room and you kiss me and say it's good."

I hugged her. "That's right." My daughter is so bright— beyond her years.

I gently explained the basics of sex. Her reaction was: "That's disgusting. When I want a baby, I'm going to the doctor to get one just like you did, Mommy."

"Dakota . . . sex or your body and the way it works is never disgusting. Babies are made through love. Love is beautiful. You know how I love you?" I wanted her to understand clearly, from the beginning.

She nodded, her eyes intent.

"I love Aunt La. That's why I am helping her have her baby, and Daddy is helping me, and so are you," I told my little daughter, who was dealing with issues well beyond her years.

Because conventional boundaries have been broken in making this decision, I wanted to explain to her what boundaries are: I had allowed my body to be used. A person can't allow their body to be used. We are expected to behave in certain ways with guidelines. Dakota had to understand the extenuating circumstances that led to this break in traditional boundaries, and this information had to be carefully restricted.

When I was a young girl and lived alone with my mother, I

was given far too much information about her life and
therefore became responsible for it in my own mind. There was
no boundary between my mother's life and my life.

My mother consulted with me before she'd make a decision.
Often before she accepted a dinner date with an admirer, she
would ask: "Shall I go for dinner with him, order a big steak
which I won't finish, and bring it home for us to share?" or
"Shall I sew Madame X's gown or refuse the money because
her body odor could knock a buzzard off a shit wagon?" We
laughed at these jokes, but the innuendos about what one has
to do for money and about my mother's sacrifices were things
I was not unaware of.

I made decisions for my mother—about her social life and
business transactions, even about our expenditures. My mother
couldn't balance our budget. I wanted my relationship with my
children to be different. I did not want to share the adult realm
of money concerns or decision making with them. I did not
want their young lives overshadowed by adult burdens, robbing
them of their childhood as Liza and I had been robbed of ours.

"I'm excited about my new cousin," Dakota said
respectfully.

"Now, when my tummy gets big and your school friends ask
if you are having a baby sister or brother, you'll tell them . . ."

"That I'm having a baby cousin." She thought a moment,
"Does Nanny know?"

"She knows, but it would make her especially glad if you
told her yourself." She did so eagerly.

Dakota was fiercely proud and protective of me, and of her
family. She came home from school telling me: "My friend
Cindy said we are silly. I told her she was jealous."

Austin picked his head up from the wall of blocks he was
building, then knocked them over with a crash. "She's jealous
because we're having a cousin and her mom isn't," he stated
in no uncertain terms.

Chapter
39

April 12, 1997

I am beginning to miss my femininity. I miss the attention on the street, polite flirting, and wine with dinner. I vaguely remember these feelings while carrying Austin, but the excitement of his arrival diminished everything else. I remember feeling beautiful with Austin. This pregnancy feels different. I am more aware of what I have given up. I don't feel desirable. Stephen constantly compliments me and makes sexual overtures, but it makes me uncomfortable. I am self-conscious in front of my husband because it is not our child that is distorting my body. I miss the freedom that naughtiness allows.

My concerns with Dakota are growing. I am not sure she feels safe enough with me to share any fears or dislikes about the pregnancy or of giving up the baby afterward. She avoids seeing me naked. Perhaps, because the pregnancy is apparent, or because it is not our baby. She might also feel embarrassed for me. I forget she is older now and has become aware of herself as a female. She prefers to be private in her bath, whereas before she would ask me to sit by the tub and tell me about her school day. Now she covers herself with a washcloth if I come in to scrub her back.

Since I am off the drugs, my tolerance levels are higher. However, too often I fall short of my expectations and become annoyed if I forget something or if I rely too much on Dakota. She tries to be so helpful, thinking how to please me and keep me undisturbed. She does her best to watch Austin and play with him so he stays out of trouble. He is a devil and she puts up with a lot. So much so that I lose sight of her age and scold her for fighting with him.

This project is much more demanding than I allowed for. I neglected the fact that I did not work full-time in either of my other pregnancies. Nor did I account for the increasing demands of my own children. I am learning to let go of little things, like not being the tough one and admitting I'm tired. I am allowing myself imperfections. My mother constantly reminded Jack and me that she could not live on a pedestal and that she was human, not without faults. I must remember not to appear faultless to my children, and to admit my shortcomings and say "I'm sorry."

I thought about my mother a lot today, much more than usual. In fact, I've been close to tears all day. She left me to deal with all the things in life she didn't want to know about: old age, death, loneliness. I am sure the anxiety regarding the upcoming amnio results and my growing frustrations with my marriage are huge contributors.

A month ago I was elated. Today I am melancholy. I was moving so quickly toward this pregnancy I didn't heed the signals of confusion and now my life seems rearranged.

It wasn't Stephen's fault that he doesn't know how to love and understand me as my mother did. I couldn't let him be who he is and relate to him as Stephen, my husband. Try as he did, I found him insufficient and it angered me.

I feel like a misfit. A misfit in my family, in society, and even in medicine. I'm expecting but not. I'm married, but I feel alone. I'm a mother with no time to enjoy her children. But, I ask myself, wasn't that the purpose of bringing this baby into the world? To break the barrier of isolation and cross back into life, to reintroduce what I have missed so desperately since my mother's death: loving, sharing, trust?

This life of mine is like swimming without getting wet. I've learned you can't love and avoid pain. I work so hard denying my feelings. I don't want to get caught blindsided by an event and emotions again. I've given myself this challenge that serves a noble purpose, yet it is quite selfish.

The first step is to bond with this baby. I must cease keeping myself detached from the incredible life growing inside me. I began this project with the intention of giving Liza's baby everything positive I have to offer—all the wonder and joy I experienced in my prior pregnancies. It can't be done without love. In just a few weeks I'll feel the baby moving inside me. I'll feel his life, and he will demand my attention as a child and not a "state of pregnancy." All or nothing is my personality and I refuse to give nothing.

I feel like an alien, lonesome to get back to my home turf, yet I don't regret what I'm doing for a second and I know after the pain is the reward.

On April 19 we received the results of the latest sonogram and all looked well. This was wonderful news. Next, we anticipated the amniocentesis, the test done to the fetus for genetic abnormalities. At that time, David and I would decide whether to be told the sex of our baby.

I received the Polaroid photo of Jen she had promised, dated April 13 . . . she was absolutely pregnant. When I removed the picture from the envelope I screamed in disbelief. The baby was growing. It was real. This was no dream. I was awake and could see my baby. I immediately called Jen. She wasn't home. I tried the office—she was out; I tried her cellular phone and was unable to get a connection. David was unavailable. I called my mother and explained the photo: "Jennifer is standing sideways in her kitchen, pointing to her stomach with a big grin on her face. She has pulled her slacks down below her belly and lifted her shirt so I could see the roundness of her." We cried.

I stopped by BBQ Restaurant, where my father was working in his office. When I showed him the picture of Jennifer, he said, " I love you, I've never seen you so happy. I'm glad you showed me the picture." I was touched by his uncharacteristic show of sentiment.

When David came home I was at the door to greet him. He, too, was awed. He kissed the picture. After dinner I talked to Jennifer.

"Wait until you see the actual belly, we've grown since then."

April 30, 1997

This morning I went to the Genetic Counseling Service in preparation for the amniocentesis that I will be having on Monday. Hearing the statistics was frightening. After the age of thirty-five, there is 1 in 150 chance of deformity and a 1 in 150 chance of complication from taking the invasive amnio test itself. (A needle is inserted into the uterus to withdraw amniotic fluid for examination.) Roughly there is 1 in 75 chance of disorder. I am overwhelmed.

Liza sent me an audiotape of her voice to play so her baby might recognize his mother's voice while inside the womb. Fable it may be, but she recorded her laugh and playful chatter about her love for him and for me. She ended the tape with lullabies which I play at night as I go to bed. Liza's voice gentles her baby, Stephen, and me to sleep each night.

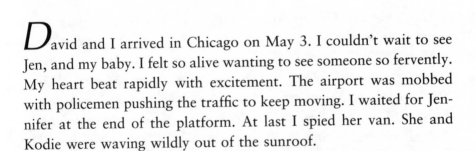

*D*avid and I arrived in Chicago on May 3. I couldn't wait to see Jen, and my baby. I felt so alive wanting to see someone so fervently. My heart beat rapidly with excitement. The airport was mobbed with policemen pushing the traffic to keep moving. I waited for Jennifer at the end of the platform. At last I spied her van. She and Kodie were waving wildly out of the sunroof.

"Jennifer," I yelled, running toward them dramatically.

I sat up front in the van with Jen. David and Kodie were in the back looking at the book we had brought her.

"Put your hand on your baby," Jen said while maneuvering her way out of the airport traffic.

I hesitated to touch her. "La." Jen laughed. "Don't be shy with me. Don't you want to feel him? It's your baby."

I put my hand on her with reluctance.

"Don't you feel he is your baby?" There was an awkward pause.

"Yes," I replied timidly. "Seeing you pregnant, Jen, knowing it's your body and my baby, I have strange and unexpected feelings . . . as if it is part of me, but not."

"This pregnancy has brought up ambiguous reactions in me also . . . but only about myself. Honestly, I know in my heart and

mind this is your child. You and I are sharing the intimacy of creation, but for me it's not the same as sharing with my husband the
making of our own child. Liza, I'm totally divorced from any feeling
of possession for this baby. I'm thrilled to do this for you and for
me. I love the baby because it's yours."

"You don't mind . . . ?" I asked, about to touch her stomach.

Jen held my hand and together we rested my palm over the baby
growing inside my cousin.

"I'm glad we were able to talk about this. It was the craziest,
unforeseen emotion, but it passed now. It came over me like a wave
and now it's gone. So, Jen, what do you think, is the baby a boy or
a girl?"

"It's a girl."

"I wonder who she'll look like. Maybe she'll have David's blue
eyes. What if she has his big thighs?"

"She could be all Wetanson, with that arrogance and tough chin."

"Or she may be a he."

"With your curly hair."

"He is so beautiful and such a wonderful mystery. I spend hours
thinking about him or her."

"Have you chosen a name?" I asked.

"If it's a girl, she will be Lilianna, and if it's a boy, either Liam
or Lucas. We will use the L for Laurie."

"I like the name Tristan."

"That's funny—I love that name. David doesn't like it."

"You could call him Tristan Luc."

"No, Jen, I want the first name to be with an 'L.' "

The weekend was strange; there seemed to be a trace of tension in
the air despite our conversation in the car, and since Stephen's
two girls were at the house, there wasn't much privacy. We bar-
becued dinner and I cleaned up while Jen put the children to bed.
Alexis and Devan had social engagements, so they were out for
the evening.

When the house was finally quiet, Stephen brought a tray of tea
from the kitchen. We sat comfortably, if not relaxed, for what would

be a discussion period, clearing up some of the many questions we had. The conversation was spontaneous.

"Let's talk about the birth," Jennifer suggested. "The doctor usually places the baby on the mother's stomach and the father cuts the umbilical cord."

I leaned forward. "The baby will be placed on your stomach, Jen, and David, I think, should cut the cord."

We all agreed.

"Then Liza will hold the baby, even before he has been cleaned or examined. She will be first to feel his birth fluids and see her baby," Jennifer said.

"Then David," Stephen said.

"Then Jen, you will hold him after David," I said.

"Agreed. Then Stephen. Any problems?"

We all smiled, searching each others faces.

"All agreed," I added in finale. Though the sequence had been stated in our legal contract, it was nice to go over it together.

"Liza, after the baby is born, do you want to bring him here when we leave the hospital?" Stephen asked.

David and I looked at each other. "Jen," I said, "what do you think? Please tell me."

"In my heart I would like you to stay with me and share the first few days, but that's not very practical and completely unhealthy. I think you'll be more comfortable staying in a hotel and getting to know your baby and how to take care of him together, without Stephen and me around."

I felt the tension leave my face. "Then we'll spend the next day here with you."

"That's the way I think it should be. If I heard the baby cry at night, instinctively I would want to go to him. My breasts secrete milk at the very sound of a baby's cry. You and David will bond with your baby." She smiled at me. "These will be moments for the three of you, alone."

It was important to specify these little details. We went over everything as if it were a rehearsal. For Jennifer in particular it was vital to lay out the steps of separation. She told me it was good for her to visualize the birth and separation and connection that would always remain between us.

May 4, 1997

Sunday crepes are a staple in the Scheu household; today was no exception. Dakota and Austin love the fanfare that surrounds Sunday breakfast; their little faces beamed with high spirits to share our tradition with Liza and David. I'm sure they relate it to the expected baby. I enjoy the exalted status I now hold in the family. It is a treat not to be the one fussing and taking care of everyone else. I smiled radiantly as they insisted I stay seated while they cleared and washed the dishes.

Today was one of the first beautiful spring mornings and I was struck with claustrophobia in the worst way. Liza and I took the car and headed to The Pea in the Pod, the maternity boutique. I thought it would be fun to shop together, but I felt unusually self-conscious about my body and how repulsed she must feel looking at me. I brought it up several times, with comments along the lines of: "Aren't you glad it's me and not you being fat."

Liza countered with: "You must hate me right now."

I hadn't thought of the position Liza was in. She who had tried so hard to get fat with pregnancy. I was doing what she longed to do, would never do. All of a sudden, for the first time, guilt raised its ugly head. For both of us. We were each showing our vulnerability and it came without warning. I apologized and so did she. We recognized the moment and moved on. I don't think we will show that lack of sensitivity again. If I feel something I'll tell her. I should have expressed my self-consciousness and she should have told me she felt guilty. My mother said we aren't perfect; this is what she meant.

We spent the remainder of the day outdoors, playing with the children and enjoying the incredible spring air. Liza and I are alike in our need to be outdoors and not waste a minute of the day.

Jennifer did not go to work Monday morning. I made some tea and brought it up to her so she could rest before our appointment with Arlene Kessler, her psychologist, whom Jennifer adored and who had asked to see us all together. Jen spoke of Arlene as her closest friend and mentor. Arlene's mother also had died of cancer. Jennifer divided the world in two parts—those who knew pain and those who did not.

What impressed me about Arlene was her well-toned sixty-year-old body. I had put her age at forty-eight. She was a handsome woman. Her brown hair was brushed softly from her angular face, revealing deep-set blue eyes that drew you to her direct gaze.

The meeting was more challenging and revealing than I'd expected. We discussed Jen's anxiety over preparing us for the change in our lives, the demands and responsibility that the birth of a child brings in its wake.

Worried as I'd been about Jen's fashion-conscious decision to wear high heels while carrying our baby, so was she worried that David and I would not adapt to parenthood. She knew our lifestyles. For me, it was long, late hours at the restaurant; David liked to have the freedom to come and go—to the theater, the gym.

"You'll see, Liza, your life will be different," Jennifer said to me.

I had no idea it caused her anguish to doubt that David and I could adjust to rearing a child. I was surprised that she thought we were unaware of the responsibilities of parenthood.

Arlene was compassionate. She pointed out to Jennifer: "If David wants to play tennis, or Liza wants to work in their garden, they'll figure it out. Everyone learns to adjust their lives in their own way."

"Yes, but they are both used to putting themselves first," said Jennifer. "Children need their parents home together, not one on duty and the other out."

David said nothing. He was waiting to hear all sides of this discussion as he did at a conference table. But I was sitting beside him and felt his body stiffen.

Jennifer rearranged herself in the chair, took a hair clip from her jacket pocket, and pulled her hair to the nape of her neck. "I know David and Liza will be great parents, but I'm edgy. It's hard to think I'll have nothing to say about the baby's upbringing, that I'll relinquish my responsibility. But that's why we're here and why I'm learning separation. The baby will always be in my life. I'm giving him to you. No one is taking him from me as my mother was taken. I was just exercising my authority."

David relaxed. Then he said, "Liza and I have a frustration to share. We don't know what to do to show our gratitude and understanding of your sacrifice. How to repay you. I know you don't want to hear it. But it's frustrating."

The psychologist looked at David and me and said firmly, "You must stop obsessing over how to show your appreciation. Showing love and sharing love is sufficient. Do you agree, Jennifer?"

"Yes," she said, turning to us, "I have no worry that you love me. It's important that we keep communicating."

"One last word on this," I said. "If you or Stephen need something from us, don't hide it. You'll let us know."

Stephen had been sitting quietly next to Jennifer on the sofa, as if the subject of the conversation, his wife's pregnancy, didn't concern him. But now he spoke. "Jennifer, you have to hear me now in front of Arlene, whom you trust. You are the most beautiful, attractive woman to me. You want me to tell you, yet when I do, you recoil. You refuse my help with your automatic I'll-do-it attitude."

Jennifer looked annoyed and moved away from him. "You admit I'm heavy. How can I be attractive?" She stood up.

"Yes, heavier, but not less lovely. That's normal when a woman is pregnant. She becomes heavier, and after, you will slim down. You haven't changed in my eyes. I respect Jennifer more than any woman. My love isn't conditional."

Arlene interrupted. "Do you hear, Jennifer?"

"I hear you," she whispered. "I'm just a little deaf." She bent over to kiss her husband.

Arlene hugged us when the session was over.

"I'll want to know all about your baby's progress, Liza and David. I've grown to care for you both through Jennifer. I want to hear about the great times to come for all of you."

I left the office feeling Arlene was our unbiased friend, and would help alleviate any tension that might arise between the Scheus and the Freilichers.

*A*fter this emotional session, we went to the hospital for the amniocentesis and further DNA testing on the baby—Jennifer, Stephen, David, and I. The four of us entered the small examining room; we are big people, and there was little room for the doctor to move about.

A nurse came in to do the ultrasound. "Do you care to learn the sex of the baby?" she asked blankly, not knowing whom to ask.

We had gone back and forth on this issue. I was just as happy not to know, since everything else had been so controlled, but lately I thought it might be wise to be prepared. I'd always wanted a girl—maybe because I liked the clothes and the long hair to braid or because of the richness of my relationship with my mother. But Stuart proved to me that a boy was wonderful, too. I saw him with his father, I saw how Mom related to Greg and Stuart, and it was equally rich. David didn't care either way. Because Jennifer felt it made a difference in how she communicated to the baby, she wanted to know the sex.

We all agreed that the decision should be the mother's. And so: "Yes," I said without hesitation. "We want to know."

At that moment, I realized that knowing the baby's sex would allow me to give him or her a name and relate to him or her as that person.

The nurse brought up the image of the fetus to the screen. I could see so clearly—the head, the legs, feet, arms, and hands. She pointed out the brain, heart, and lungs. Everything looked perfect. We were all thrilled and relieved.

"It looks like a boy," she said.

"*A boy.*" The scream went up from all of us in unison.

"A boy. I can't believe it." It suddenly seemed so real the fact that we were having a son. I could see him.

Jen was screaming. "It's a boy. What are we going to name him? When are you going to name him?"

Stephen wanted a better look at his penis.

We looked at the sonogram for a long while, watched our son kicking his feet. He looked happy, too, as if he were saying hello to us.

The nurse laughed as he looked at the screen. "Definitely a boy."

We saw him suck his thumb. He was sucking with one hand and covering his mouth with the other.

"He'll probably be a thumb sucker like you, La," Jen said. "I hope he'll stop before he's twenty-one."

We were laughing as the doctor came in.

"Can you make room for me?" she asked cheerfully. She knew the situation. We pressed together to make space while she explained the process of inserting a needle through the stomach into the uterus and withdrawing the fluid from the amniotic sac in which the fetus floats. I looked at Jennifer skeptically as the nurse suggested we not watch.

Jen squeezed my hand. "I've had this done before, it's not fun."

I watched the sonograph screen and saw the needle penetrate the sac and withdraw several vials of fluid. The doctor was careful not to touch the fetus with the needle, and I held my breath as she worked. The whole procedure looked too close to me, but the baby seemed unperturbed. It was over quickly, and as always, Jennifer was a trooper, although she did look pale. We would know all but two of the test results in a couple of days; the other test results took three weeks. The DNA test had been done on the five of us.

After we paid our bill, the nurse gave me a green diaper bag filled with baby formula, powder, lotion, magazines on child care, and a book on birthing. I never thought I would actually own one of these. It was my first baby gift.

"Okay," Jen said as we were leaving the hospital. "You have to name this kid so I can start calling him by his name."

"Let's spread the news," I said. We called my mother and Greg, then David's parents. Their reaction was pure joy.

My father said, "Now we have another restaurateur."

"No way," I insisted. "We'll let him decide."

I spent the flight home deciding between "Lucas" and "Liam." By the time we landed, I had changed my mind a dozen times.

Waiting for the results of the amniocentesis was unnerving, especially since we had seen our healthy baby boy. I jumped every time the phone rang on Wednesday, expecting it to be Jennifer with the test results. I was out of breath all day. She called me at Sambuca at three o'clock in the afternoon. "Hold on, I have David on the other line. Everything is fine."

I felt an ache leave my body, and a most welcome warm flood of contentment replace it. I hoped Jennifer would experience this release of her pain after the baby is born.

By Illinois law the mother/child relationship can be determined by the same tests that apply to the father/child relationship. In other words, the DNA test, which all of us had done, including the fetus, was appropriate to establish that the woman who bore the child was *not* the natural and therefore legal mother and in fact this child was genetically ours.

Based on this law, Stephen's father, Ralph, who is a Chicago attorney, had prepared a petition in which the four of us jointly asked the court to declare David and me the legal and natural parents of the baby; Stephen and Jennifer would not be considered natural parents. This was the first time such an order was entered in Illinois. As we prayed, it went through without a further hearing. We sent Northwestern Memorial Hospital certified copies of the orders before Jennifer's admission for the birth. We thought we had all our bases covered.

May 10, 1997, was my first Mother's Day. I received cards and phone calls. Mom and Jen sent me a lilac bush to grow in my garden.

The best Mother's Day gift for me and my mother was Jen's call to tell us that the hospital had reported that the final amnio test had come back negative.

"Everything is perfect, La, like we saw him to be. Happy Mother's Day, La La . . . give me his name."

"Now that we know everything is fine, I think now we can focus on his name."

At dusk, when the flurry of people were gone and there were no more phone calls and gifts, I went outside on the porch. I sat next to the sculpture of my grown baby bird and let my eyes take in the open field before me. The earth had been turned and newly planted, but the shoots of green beans were not yet visible. The air was warm and sweet-scented. Soon I would have my baby. I was truly a mother this day, a member of the most revered group in the world. Membership in it is lifelong.

David came outside and sat on the bench beside me. We were quiet. It felt so peaceful, sitting hand in hand with my husband, having no need to talk.

I rested my head on his shoulders. "Luc, just Luc."

"Luc," he said, gazing off at the smoke from the passing train that looked like a toy in the distance.

"Luc. Our son. That's his name. Yes?"

"Luc Freilicher."

I thought of my baby bird and his stamina. The last time I had seen him, he was as large as a full-grown pigeon and had a fuzzy yellow head. What a miracle it was that that little thing survived out there on my air conditioner. He was so independent, brave, and strong.

June 10, 1997

Memorial Day weekend has passed. The three days at home with my family has allowed me a glimpse of how wonderfully crazy our life together is. We had no social plans and spent each day dealing with errands and enjoying each other's company. Austin is in the throes of terrible threes, with his motto—"because I want to"—being echoed after every crisis. Decorating the walls and doors with crayon scribble was his latest project. It is hard to channel him and not break his spirit; he is such an energetic and inquisitive child.

Luc is kicking more often, a gentle reminder that we are in this together: me, Luc, Liza, and Mommy.

The seventh anniversary of Mommy's death came and went May 30. Surprisingly, I was in a good mood most of the day and felt truly closer to her living spirit—rather than being preoccupied by the specifics of her death. Carrying Luc feels like she is here with me. The extreme sadness is being replaced by the joy of feeling Luc grow.

Stanley remembered the anniversary and we spoke. Everyone in the family called except Jack. I left a message on his machine. It went unanswered.

I was hurt. I would have felt better sharing with my brother

*the closeness of memories. I was thinking how happy we all
were driving cross-country, how untouchable we felt laughing
and singing together. But Jack was angry. He turned away from
the reality of Mommy's illness; he wouldn't acknowledge her
death even to comfort me.*

*I am at the halfway mark of my pregnancy. The last ultrasound
was on May 30th. Luc's heart is perfectly formed now and we
have no real reason to worry about his health. He is most
definitely David's child. No matter how the doctor prods him
to change position, he lies back calmly. Liza and I would have
kicked violently; I hope he has some of our sass.*

*This week Liza wrestled with the problem of installing a
washer/dryer to accommodate her expanding family, while I
wrestled with new bras to accommodate my expanding body.*

*Dakota returned home from a weekend at Hilary's home in
Michigan with the request to spend the coming weekend again
with Hilary and her pal Michael [Hilary's son]. Both Stephen
and Hilary were shocked when I agreed.*

*"Are you going to be okay without her for so long a time?"
Stephen asked.*

*"I'm not that fragile. Of course she can go." I couldn't let
my attachment to my mother be replaced by an unhealthy
attachment to my daughter. I want her to be free.*

*My days are becoming more difficult. The weight of Luc's
maturing body keeps me from sleeping soundly. The days are
long and tiring. I experienced my first migraine headache. I am
retaining water and my ankles are swelling. Another in the list
of firsts for me in this pregnancy. Dr. Isola says it is because I
am older now.*

*Father's Day is next weekend. Time is moving quickly.
Stephen is back in my graces since that eye-opening session
with Arlene. He has been caring and affectionate to me in spite
of our distant sexual love affair. I truly revere his
nonjudgmental attitude and feel loved and nurtured. I have
been working to catch myself from blaming Stephen for my*

miseries and look to his strengths. I thought I needed no one but my mother, which was wrong. I do need my husband and the love and support of a man for a woman. These feelings have been long absent, and I am loving, loving him.

I cried myself to sleep last night with violent heart-wrenching sobs as I haven't done in years. I hadn't felt well all day. Stephen picked me up at the office early; we dropped Baci off at the vet for his checkup and inoculations and stopped for a light dinner so I would not have to cook. Before going home we collected Baci and rented a film at the video store. I chose The Bridges of Madison County.

We went to bed early. Austin snuggled awhile and Stephen carried him to his own bed. Kodie finished her homework, came in for a kiss, and went to bed.

Stephen and I settled down to watch the film. I saw my mother in the movie everywhere. Not because of any similarity in lifestyle, more because of [the character] Francesca's death and her children's discovery of her other life. The movie is about love and loss. And although I cried for the characters, it sparked hidden tears of grief, loneliness, and pain for my mother's passing. More than that, it terrified me to think I might feel this way again when Luc is born.

June 19, 1997

Liza and David came to spend the weekend with us free of medical or legal duties. We missed each other and Liza missed Luc. Also, today was David's forty-forth birthday. Double digits are good luck and he couldn't be more thankful or happy for what this year will bring. I was feeling particularly connected to David; he is a sobering presence for me. Perhaps it's his experience with guiding people toward sensible decisions in his business. We were in the living room after breakfast reading the newspaper when I gave in to instinct. "David, would you like to feel your baby kick, even listen to him? This is your baby. Share his growth with me." David is cerebral, and reserved when it comes to sharing affection. "Come on, put your head on my stomach."

He put down the paper and looked quizzically at Stephen, who appeared to accept the gesture as normal. The four of us are so at ease with each other, this is not an invasion of marital intimacy.

"Your son is kicking persistently in salutation to your

birthday. Sit here on the floor in front of me and put your head on this big pillow." I patted my tummy, "Enjoy him."

"Really?" he asked, almost shyly. It was very endearing.

"Really," I replied, and couldn't help but smile. He looked like an innocent teenager, not a corporate executive.

I was seated on the sofa. David sat on the floor and rested his head against my stomach. I kept my hands at my sides so as not to touch him and make him self-conscious. This union was between father and son.

A smile spread across his face. "Oh, he kicked my cheek. Liza, come here, you must feel this with me."

The parents of the baby inside me shared the wonders of his early life movements together as parents do. At this time they were rapt in their dream come true and not even aware of Stephen and me.

The next day Stephen and Liza rearranged my garden while David weeded, and I took care of the kids. Liza's energy for gardening is so like my mother's. She's such a different Liza than she was a year ago—open and loving. I'm proud of her, and in some way I know that I helped in this transformation. We are alike in determination and spirit.

"Mom, have you seen Baci?" Kodie asked, coming around the house. "He's not in the house or in the backyard." She had been helping Stephen and Liza pull up bushes; her sweatshirt and jeans were covered in dirt.

"I haven't seen him. Baci . . . Baci . . ." I called down the street. "That dog is always chasing squirrels."

"Oh no, here comes that awful Mrs. Cooper," Kodie said, pushing her long braids behind her back in readiness for a confrontation.

"Mrs. Cooper is a retired schoolmarm, who idles her time canvassing the neighborhood with a critical eye, looking for trouble and finding enemies. She lives on the cul-de-sac," I explained to Liza.

Kodie began to giggle and sing a ditty: "Cooper, snooper, doggy pooper."

"Hush, that's not funny," I scolded, but snickered with her.

"*Are you looking for your mutt?*" inquired the primly dressed woman: a pleated plaid skirt, loafers, and an oatmeal-colored sweater set. Her voice had a threatening timbre. "*He's digging in my garden again. I'm warning you . . .*"

Stephen put down his spade, and came prepared to be mediator. "*Kodie, run down and get Baci.*"

She took the red dog leash from the doorknob and raced down the block calling, "*Baci . . . Baci.*"

"*Would anyone care for some iced tea?*" I asked as a gesture to keep the peace.

"*No, dear,*" said Mrs. Cooper, noting my enlarged figure and smiling up at Stephen. "*When is your baby due, Mr. Scheu?*"

Stephen grinned. "*Oh, it's not my baby. It's his.*" He pointed to David, who looked up from his weeding to nod acknowledgment as Liza walked over, hugging him with showy affection.

Kodie came back with Baci.

Mrs. Cooper pulled her sweater around her.

Stephen went on to explain that I was the gestational carrier for Liza and David.

She flushed, believing, I'm sure, it was some incestuous affair. "*How could you let your wife do such a thing? Who do you people think you are to play God?*"

Her indignation caused the color to rise from her neck.

Stephen loved to cause this flurry; it was his favorite joke, but the insinuations it aroused enraged me. I was furious. "*And who are you to imply he can control me?*"

Mrs. Cooper coughed and sidled away. "*Keep your dog at home,*" she called over her shoulder.

We barely heard her, we were laughing so hard.

Late at night Dakota woke up and came into our room all puffy from sleep. She got in bed with Stephen and me and reached toward me to snuggle, with the sweetest smile on her lips. "*Mommy, does your life ever seem like a dream that goes on forever and each day gets better?*"

I lay there lost in her little-girl scent. I love her so completely

*and dangerously I constantly resist being selfish with her time.
She murmured on in a soft voice, half-asleep. "I'm the luckiest
of my friends, Mommy, they're all jealous of me."*

"Why are they jealous, Kodie?"

"Because you're my best friend."

"Kodie?"

She was sleeping.

*"How lucky I am to have you," I whispered to my sleeping
child.*

*Sunday afternoon Stephen drove Liza and David to the airport.
It was hard for them to leave us. I stayed home, and as I
watched Kodie prepare a salad and make hamburger patties
that Stephen would later barbecue, I reflected on our short time
together. It was a time of coupling. I think we all moved even
closer, allowing ourselves to accept each other as individuals.*

*I don't remember feeling this pain-free in the longest time.
Wonderful things seem to be multiplying from this one act of
love. I feel free of fear: fear of loss, fear of being alone, and
fear of not being important after the baby is born. I haven't
felt this secure in love since my childhood. It is hard to face
the truth of letting go. I hope I can hold on to this lesson I so
purposely set out to learn and teach my children: not to be
timid about making a commitment of love.*

*I saw Dr. Isola this morning. I think she takes special interest
in this baby. After the examination, she spends extra time with
me asking about my own expectations and takes personal pride
in Luc's growth. I got a letter from her telling me to limit my
work time to six hours a day. All the exhaustion and pressure
I feel on my bladder is just a fact of life—I'm not as young as
I used to be.*

July 25, 1997

"How do you feel about me getting a vasectomy?" Stephen asked while driving to work. I was surprised that he mentioned it, and had been fearful to suggest it myself, thinking he would think it would emasculate him. I know it is the right decision for us. I have no desire, beyond Liza's and David's happiness and my healing, for a child. I am content with this being the finale of my reproductive life. Stephen has enough financial obligations to his four children. We have weathered the storm that rocked the foundation of our marriage and now I look forward to the return of a close intimate relationship with my husband. I agreed to the vasectomy.

I have officially entered the uncomfortable stage of pregnancy: beyond the heat and humidity is the unending pressure of the baby's weight and constant kicking.

The workload in the office is mounting. Though leaving early at three o'clock in the afternoon has been a relief, I am unable to manage all the problems that arise daily. Last night Stephen had dinner alone in town while he waited for me to *finish at nine o'clock, trying to stay on top of things. I wish I could take the stance that, due to circumstances, I didn't care if I fell behind, but my pride prohibits that. I would feel no differently if the child I'm carrying were my own. Often I feel faint and this afternoon I fell at the office and had to lie down. My boss realized this could become a liability to the company and decided to put me on disability leave right away. I felt guilty when he told me. I also felt disposable. I know I deserve this time at home, but I don't want to shirk my responsibilities.*

I promised Ellen, my assistant, that I would help out from home until the office got up to speed. I packed every pending piece of business as well as my personal things and left, feeling sad, knowing I'd miss Ellen and the rest of the staff.

Stephen and my children responded to my early departure from work with enthusiasm. I haven't been a nonworking mom in a while and wondered if I will be successful.

Kodie and Austin have gotten used to me not doing what I ordinarily do. I pamper myself, almost to obsession, avoiding any exertion or roughhousing. Gratefully Christine has the stamina for Austin's many chase schemes. A remaining consideration is Stephen, who justly complains about losing his sexual partner. I told him, not in anger but in decisive tones, that I will not jeopardize this pregnancy in any way. I didn't tell him that I have absolutely no desire.

"I'll remain celibate until the baby is born; unfortunately I have to impose the same condition on you. Sex can wait . . . and no extramarital activity is allowed. Remember we have a legal contract with Liza and David. We'll sue you," I teased, trying to be humorous but failing grievously. In truth I am becoming more and more nervous approaching Luc's birth.

I have rehearsed and visualized the entire scenario in my head. But what about my heart? Can I control the most overpowering of emotions? I love Luc. I've sustained him, sung him to sleep, felt his life inside me. Can I control my heart? I believe I can. I think of Mommy being snatched away from

me. I will be different with Luc. He will always be in my life.
I wonder how my body will react, if hormones will be stronger
than my mind over this matter? I am anxious for this to be
over. I wonder how tough I really am. The speed at which we
are approaching the baby's birth is frightening.

I had researched all cribs and gone from choosing wood to wrought
iron and back to wood. The wrought iron is gorgeous but difficult
to open. I finally ordered a classic white, four-poster wood crib and
bureau for the New York nursery. For the Long Island nursery Max
gave me the crib she used for Stuart and Sophia. It, too, was white
and in perfect condition. So now I had two cribs. My mother and I
combed all the department stores, baby boutiques, and catalogs
looking at the unending selection of bedding patterns. For the city
I chose blue pale yellow and ecru checks on quilted piqué cotton for
curtains, bumpers, and the dust ruffle. The country nursery would
be more casual, a sunny plaid of yellow and apple green. It was fun
picking everything out, discussing it with Jen and my mother. I
found a small chest of drawers at a tag sale and sanded it down and
painted it white with trim to match the plaid, and put that in the
house. Mom and Joe made whimsical paintings for the walls. The
two nurseries were waiting for Luc.

I began planning for Jennifer's visit in August. She was coming
with Kodie and Austin and Stephen and his daughters for two
weeks. A houseful. Mom and Greg were organizing a baby shower
for me and Jen on August 16th. It would be held at my house and
Greg was going to make all the food himself. Mom and I made up
the guest list and sent out the invitations, which read: *Please come*
to a baby shower for Liza Freilicher honoring Jennifer Scheu. This
would be a long-awaited opportunity for me to proclaim to Jennifer
my love and esteem in the presence of people who admired us and
wished us well. Oh, if only I could have draped her in garlands of
laurels like a triumphant warrior.

I was glad that Jennifer was at home and able to relax. Her work
schedule had been enough to wear anyone out, and being pregnant,
keeping to that demanding pace was heroic.

I thought back on how Jen and I had evolved through our growing years, what turns our lives had taken and how they had changed us. Over time and through separations, we had come to know one another in the deepest sense of the word. For that I thank our mothers. Jennifer, who was timid, was now bold. And me? Perhaps because of my profession and the necessity of mingling with people, I was self-confident. Maybe all people are alike, each having an Achilles' heel and each finding his own way to become courageous.

David and I prepared for Jennifer's arrival. We sanded down our paint-peeled collectibles, repainted and polyurethaned them. There were no stylish paint flakes anywhere to endanger the children. To make space at the house, I emptied closets, which were ample but sparsely filled. I lined shelves and drawers and fixed anything that was broken. All drawers slid easily and the fence gate swung so you no longer had to lift it to close.

I figured out what to give Jen as a fun shower gift: a new gym bag filled with exercise clothing, sweatshirts, shoes, socks, deodorant, foot spray, Evian water, sweat towel, and a gift certificate for a year's membership to the health club of her choice. She was anxious to get back into shape as soon as the baby was born. At least she'd have something fun to open while I opened my shower gifts.

Chapter
45

August 8, 1997

*Today is the first day of our vacation. I am looking forward
to spending a day with my father. I'll take Liza's Jeep, which
she left for me, upstate to my mother's house. Stanley won't
be there. I'll be alone with my mommy. I used to be aching
with grief at that house, where happy memories accented her
absence. The house is still warm with her smell. I had found
myself looking for her, expecting to see her, hear her call out
to me. At the house I am surrounded by her essence. I have no
fears or hesitation this time. My mother is inside of me; I don't
have to look for her. Often I fantasize about the relationship
my mother would have had with Dakota and Austin—all of us
being her children. This is a great loss and I envy Liza for what
she will have with her mother and Luc.*

DAVID AND I WERE on the porch of the house Thursday morning
waiting for Jennifer and Stephen and the kids. I was in my summer
attire. David took pictures of me showing a sunlit smile beneath a

straw floppy-brimmed hat, my hair pulled back in a ponytail, now almost to my waist. My daily costume was cutoff denim shorts and a tank top, so I could feel the heat of the sun on my arms and legs.

They arrived at noon and piled out of the Jeep. Stephen's height always impressed me. Jennifer was in her seventh month, full-blown pregnant and beautiful in a black minidress. Alexis and Devan, too, were tall like their father. Austin and Kodie came out of the car last. Kodie was a dainty, lithe little girl who was already showing signs of the woman she'd become. She took Austin by the hand and led him into the house.

We got them situated. Devan and Alexis were in the downstairs bedroom, Jen and Stephen in the upstairs guest room, and Kodie and Austin were in the nursery on twin beds I borrowed from my neighbor. After they were comfortable, I suggested we sit outside by the pool. The temperature was nearly ninety degrees.

"Jen, there are chaises out there. Lie down and relax. I have lunch ready."

"I'll help you. I have to make Austin his cheese sandwich."

"Let me do it. Lie down, you had a long drive. Was there much traffic?"

"Not bad. Kodie gets turkey. I brought all the cold cuts. Where do you want lunch, outside or on the porch?"

"The porch is cooler. I made salad for us and plain broiled chicken for the kids."

"Austin won't eat that. Stephen, please watch them while I help Liza."

Lunch was hectic, everyone eating something different. The girls were impatient to go swimming. Austin was running in and out, slamming the screen door, and Jennifer was calling after him not to dig in the garden or to open the gate.

"Everything is childproof. He can't get in the pool area or open the gate. I've enclosed all of the backyard with a fence," I said, bringing a salad of fresh mozzarella cheese, home-grown tomatoes and basil.

"Can I be excused?" asked Devan, who had taken a bite out of her lunch and left the picked-over remains on her plate.

Alexis got up with her and went out to the pool.

"Jen, sit down, you haven't eaten anything."

"Wait till you have children, you'll have to change your continental ways. They eat early and fast. I have a ton of laundry to do," Jennifer said, exchanging glances with her husband as if to say, "What does she know about family and children?" "My mother's washing machine wasn't working, so I have a three-day load. Your washer is upstairs, isn't it?"

"I'll do it for you. Let's just sit together and finish our lunch. Was it hard for you to be at your mother's? Did Stanley come up?"

The door slammed, Jennifer jumped, and Kodie came in wearing a wet bathing suit that dripped onto the floor. "Where's my clay, Mommy? I want to make a sculpture for Nannie."

"I'll get it." Jen pulled herself heavily out of the chair. "Don't go in the house with that wet suit, Kodie."

"Jen, please tell me where the clay is. Don't climb the stairs," I said.

"No, I have to put the wash in anyway." She was already out of the room.

For all my planning I couldn't get Jennifer to leave a thing for me to do. Was she being perversely independent, did she think I was incompetent? The more I tried to assist, the more adamantly she pushed me aside. I promised myself this would be a time of family interaction. She was caring for my child, I wanted with all my heart to care for her and her family. It should have been a time for fun; it was supposed to be Jen's vacation.

I set Kodie up with clay at the glass dinner table, with a towel on the chair so she wouldn't get the cushion wet. Austin came in, also dripping wet.

"I want to do that, too," he said, and moved a chair next to Kodie.

"Wait, Austin, let me give you a towel." I picked up a towel from the floor that one of the kids had dropped.

He sat down before I got it under him. I had to lift him up and dry him off and the seat. Kodie gave him a wad of clay.

"I want what you have," he said, grabbing at Kodie's beginnings of a horse.

Where I had hoped for harmony there was discord.

Austin started to cry as Jennifer came onto the porch. There were beads of perspiration on her forehead and her face was flushed.

"Mommy, I tried to keep him quiet. He doesn't listen," Kodie announced as she attempted to repair her clay horse.

"I'll take him. Thanks, Kodie-girl. Sorry, Liza, he's a devil. This is a difficult age," Jennifer said as her son hugged her knees.

Were I a maestro, I'd have tapped gently with my baton and begun a symphony to serenade Jennifer where she dozed beneath the poolside umbrella or lounged on the porch. I wanted to treat her like a queen.

The vacation had only begun, but it was not going as I'd envisioned. It was awkward; there was a lot of tension that neither of us vocalized. For me it was frustration and annoyance that Jennifer wouldn't let me treat her as I had planned. Pampering her would have been an outlet for me, a way of expressing my gratitude and my love. It would have been my opportunity to show her without words.

Jennifer, I imagined, regarded me as one with a lingering naivete, with no idea of what life in the real world of children was about. She wouldn't say it to me, though, not after our session with Arlene. She was supposed to let David and me become parents in our own way, but I was sure she confided her critical assessments to her husband.

The next morning I woke up early. The house was quiet. I tiptoed downstairs, thinking everyone was asleep. To my surprise, Jennifer was at the kitchen stove, Kodie and Austin were at the table waiting for their next batch of pancakes, and Devan and Alexis were doing laps in the pool. "Hi," Jen said. "I made coffee for you."

"Thanks," I responded weakly. I had wanted to make breakfast for them. It was frustrating; she wouldn't allow me to be a hostess. "You didn't have to make coffee."

"Stephen drinks it; David too, doesn't he? You don't all have to suffer that with me. I'm fine with tea. Liza, what do you think if we paint the baby's bathroom. I know you are superstitious, but this kid is going to be here soon and you need to get ready."

"Jen, you can't paint pregnant," I said.

"Okay, but let me help, remember when we painted Sambuca together!"

"It'll be beautiful, but all you'll do is supervise. We'll have it done in two hours."

"And I can mix the paint."

Stephen came downstairs and poured himself a cup of coffee. He heard our conversation and said, "I'll go buy the paint."

We did the job in three hours, with all four kids watching. I was on the stepladder painting downward from the ceiling with straight strokes. Jen handed me brushes loaded with the paint she'd mixed according to her own recipe for an antique glaze. We were working in good rhythm in the bathroom when the phone rang.

"Someone . . . Alexis . . . can you get it?" I called.

"Hello," I heard her say. "One minute, she's painting. Liza, it's Bonni; she says it's important."

"Can't I call her back?"

"No, she's taking her son to the doctor."

"What is it? I can't get off the ladder, we're squeezed in here."

"She says she can't come to the shower because Ryan has a fever and an earache."

"I'm sorry. Tell her we'll miss her and to get him better. That's most important. I'll call her tomorrow."

"Bonni says she's sorry and sends love to you both."

"Thanks, Alexis. Jen . . . I have to finish the ceiling, then we're done."

Jennifer handed me a fresh brush. "That's not right of Bonni not to come. Why couldn't her husband stay home with Ryan?"

"I'm sure she'd have arranged it if she could have. Never mind. We'll have tons of people."

"She's your best friend." She shrugged.

I ignored what seemed like an expression of hurt and anger. Painting the bathroom had given me and Jen an opportunity to do something together, something that recalled an earlier innocent time in our lives.

By lunchtime the paint was dry, the towels hung on the racks, and my mother's watercolors hung on the walls.

After everyone was fed lunch, Jen and I went to Hildreth's, the local country department store, to look at a bookshelf I wanted for Luc's room. Neither of us had the courage to initiate a conversation about the awkwardness we were feeling. When we came home I sat down and wrote her a long letter expressing my pent-up feelings: that I recognized we were both being controlling and that we were not in competition with each other. After I read it, I tore it up, afraid my displeasure might offend her.

The Saturday morning of the party the temperature had reached ninety-two degrees before noon. The air conditioner kept the house cool, but I had planned to entertain my guests outside on the porch. I opened the doors and put on the overhead fan to push the cooler air to the outside.

Jennifer arranged the blue-and-white paper plates on the big glass table for a buffet. I swept the porch and picked flowers for every room. Greg said he'd bring the platters of sandwiches and salads by three-thirty. The company was due at four o'clock, after everyone, presumably, returned from the beach. I went upstairs for a fast shower. Jennifer went to her room to lie down before her shower.

At three o'clock, my friend Mindy called to tell me she would not be coming to the baby shower. I understood. Mindy had lost a baby in her fifth month and was undergoing fertility treatments; it would be emotionally difficult for her to attend the shower. She said her husband, Glen, would stop by and drop off the gifts she'd gotten for Jen and me. It was not so long ago I felt the way Mindy must have been feeling when I looked at the women pushing baby carriages through the park, as if that happiness was out of reach to me. How strongly our lives are governed by emotion and how quickly the pendulum swings between happiness and sadness. Jennifer and I were being guided in this pilgrimage by emotion—she to escape misery and I to find a joy I had never known.

Joe and my mother arrived early. Joe took the Jeep to town to pick up the one hundred blue helium balloons he'd ordered to tie to the fence and cover the ceiling of the porch. The ceiling fan blew them about festively. Mom went into the kitchen to make pitchers of fresh lemonade with mint I had picked from my garden. At three-thirty, I began to look for Greg. The four kids came down, all of them excited. Jen had swept her thick blond hair up off her neck, leaving a few loose wisps that gave her an ethereal quality. She wore high-heeled white sandals and a gauzy white Empire sundress that fell softly below her knees. To me she looked like a mythical goddess of fertility.

I was wearing a T-shirt and flowered short skirt. I had been dieting since I stopped the fertility drugs and had lost fifteen pounds.

The first guests to arrive were Rachel and her mother Marie. Rachel and Jen had gone to high school together in New York. Rachel had been Jen's companion during her disco days, when she danced on top of the loudspeakers. Rachel's body was still taut and athletic. Her mother, Marie, who was born in France, spoke to Jen in French and Jen answered in French; the three of them sat down together. Other guests drove out from New York City and from Long Island. Still, no Greg. I was getting nervous. My father called and said he couldn't come. He was competing in an important automobile race today and was at the Limerock track in Connecticut. Erica and Jack had also found reasons not to come.

At last Greg pulled up. The expressway had been bumper to bumper with beach traffic. He and Max brought in mountains of cocktail sandwiches, all beautifully garnished with the crusts cut off. Stuart carried in bowls of potato salad and crudités with dip. I looked at Jen. She was still talking to Rachel and Marie. Sophia found Austin and they began to play together with his toy truck. Stuart refused to let him have his matchbox car, so an incipient battle had to be defused. Jen and Stephen gave each other knowing looks, showing their disapproval of Stuart and of Greg and Max as disciplinarians.

Stanley arrived with his wife, Vivian, a tall redhead, very vivacious. He looked subdued. Vivian plunged into boisterous greetings. They sat on the couch together as if we were distant friends rather than family. Stanley and Jennifer were chatting socially when Vivian asked him to get her some wine. That was the last I saw of Jen and

Stanley together. She sat alone on a chair next to Kodie and held her hand. Her eyes glazed over with tears.

"Jen. What's the matter?" I rushed to ask her.

"I just wish Mommy were here. All at once I feel like I'm a stranger."

"This party is for you. Everyone who came, came primarily to honor you. Remember what you said. Remember your vision, Jen. Your mother is with us." She wiped her eyes and nodded.

Everyone ate and congratulated us and then asked me to open my gifts: little-boy clothes, carriage blankets, everything for my new baby. Max gave me a basket full of layette items, which I didn't even know I needed.

With this shower, our baby, our unique closeness and endeavor had become a public affair. Our friends felt honored to take part. The gifts were given to both of us out of admiration and joy. My friends, who hadn't known Jennifer well before, now loved her.

Jen received a gift certificate to Elizabeth Arden. When I gave her the gym bag, she hooted with pleasure and my mother gave her an oil painting she had done of a little boy looking at a vase of flowers.

"I'll hang it in my entrance hall," Jen said, wiping her tear-filled eyes.

I saw my friend Steven Donziger, who'd gone to American University when Jen and I were there. Steven has an incredible mind, is a political writer, attorney, and sometime adventurer who travels to the world's revolutionary hot spots. On top of that, he is tall and handsome. He and Jennifer went off to sit in a corner and talk. She no longer looked forlorn.

After the shower, when everyone left, Greg and Max remained. Alexis took the younger children to play upstairs.

We adults sat on the porch amid baby clothes and toys and piles of overstuffed boxes. Max kicked off her sandals and put her long tan legs on the sofa over Greg's knees. He was looking dreamy, filled with emotion. He just looked at Jen and me and soaked it in. Jennifer took her hair down and went to lie on the opposite sofa. I brought her a cold wet cloth to wipe the perspiration from her face. It was seven o'clock and still so hot and humid. Stephen and David pulled over the heavy iron chairs from the table and joined the group. I, of course, was picking up bits of wrapping paper that had escaped the trash can.

"So, let's gossip," Max said.

We laughed. "That's the best part of a party," Jen said, her eyes closed.

We talked about everyone, what they were up to, how they'd worn their hair, what they were wearing, who looked older. Jen hadn't seen my friend Amy since high school. She had three kids. Jen couldn't believe how gorgeous she looked.

Jen mentioned the imminence of the baby's arrival and Greg got up to feel Luc kick. Max, to whom mothering is a serious matter, filled with vital decisions, had just faced the vaccine issue with three-year-old Sophia. She asked me what inoculations I would give Luc. The conversation became serious. Max suggested I explore my options regarding vaccines. "There are things you should learn about," she stated, and proceeded to cite chapter and verse.

While she was speaking, Jennifer remained quiet, then suddenly she pulled herself up off the sofa and abruptly walked out of the room giving Max a wicked look.

Maxine sensed Jen's anger. "I only said . . ." she began to protest, and her eyes filled with tears. I could see how stunned she was by Jennifer's hasty exit. It angered her that she couldn't defend herself.

There was no time to intervene. Stephen went after his wife. The episode happened so quickly I could barely fathom what exactly had transpired. David looked bewildered. He went over to Max, but she shrugged him away.

Greg said in a low voice, "She wanted to contribute. Luc is important to us also."

Max went to the powder room. I heard the water running, but it didn't obliterate her sobs. When she came out, she and Greg collected their children and left without further comment. Max's eyes were red, and she moved swiftly. I had never seen her so upset.

The incident was no one's fault, but I was afraid it would cause a rift between me and Jen and Greg and Max. I didn't know from whom the apology should come. There was no harm meant. None at all. "I'm sorry," I said as they left.

Jennifer was crying when I knocked on her bedroom door. "Come in," she sobbed.

"Jen, what happened?"

"Max has no business telling us what shots Luc should get."

"She meant no harm. She is concerned. She did a lot of research when it was time to inoculate Sophia. She wasn't telling us what to do."

"Who is she to advise, as if she knows it all?"

"Jen. She was just trying to be helpful."

"I'm tired. Look how swollen my feet are. Stephen will put the kids to bed," she said dismissively.

As we said good night, I felt helpless and I knew Greg and Max felt awful. I was sorry. Jen had misunderstood Max's intention. I suspected it was a result of the prevailing tension that had become so strong over the past week.

I didn't hear Jennifer get up the next morning. The four children had had breakfast and she was making pancakes for Stephen when I came downstairs at eight A.M. From then on, for two endless days, there was a wall between us. Jennifer, I felt, make a point of avoiding any private time with me. She was always occupied with the kids, and even seized any chance she could get to go out marketing. Also, she spent hours on her computer.

"Writing my journal," she explained.

"Do you want to talk about it?" I asked.

"No, not now. I want to finish this."

I would have liked to peek over her shoulder. I felt like a character in the Japanese movie, *Rashomon,* where three individuals share a dramatic experience together but have radically different versions of what exactly occurred. I wondered what Jennifer's version of the baby shower would be like.

The morning of the Scheus' departure was hurried.

"We have a plane to catch," Jen announced, and went bustling off.

Stephen brought down their bags and David helped him pack the van.

I tried to find a moment to speak to Jennifer alone and get her to tell me what she thought transpired. I wanted to hold her close; she seemed so distant. I was afraid. I had a pain in my heart that only fear brings. It was the end of August. I wouldn't be with Jen until it was time for Luc's birth. I couldn't allow her to leave while this meaningless obstacle remained between us.

"Let's go," Stephen called, and whisked Jennifer into the car. All at once, it seemed, David and I were kissing them good-bye. The usual sadness we felt at their departure was not there. None of what Jen or I had anticipated had happened. I didn't know what had happened or why. When the car turned out of the driveway, I began to cry.

I had been abandoned. Jennifer was being driven away with my baby and I was left unneeded, unloved, and unable to reach them. What was she thinking? How was she feeling carrying the burden of Luc?

I watched the clock all day, minute by minute, until the sun went down and I knew she was again in Chicago. When I got her on the phone, I was barely able to hear her voice over the noise of their arrival. Baci was barking, the children were tired and crying, and Stephen was calling out orders.

"We had a safe trip. All of us. Luc slept. It's okay, La. Don't worry. I'm tired and I'm glad to be home. I thought about it on the plane. We were each trying so hard to help the other, we knocked each other over. I'm going to sleep. I'll speak to you tomorrow." She hung up. Her voice, though tired, conveyed the same warmth I remembered from before this awful episode.

I felt better, but we still had to talk. I wondered about Jennifer's perception of this time together.

Chapter
46

August 12 and 23, 1997

The week at Liza's was different than I imagined. I'm sure she was stretched to the limit with a house full of four children, especially the demands of Austin, a precocious three-year-old. I tried to relax and allow the closeness we shared long distance to take over, but the affection seemed tenuous at best. I would like to be able to record in this journal some conversations, exchanges of feeling between us, but there were none. Each of us was busy keeping our own lives out of each other's hair. I expected Liza and David to want to touch my stomach more, be more aware of the strain on my body. I believe pregnancy is one of those things you can't understand unless you have lived through it. She does, however, try to protect my time to relax, which is totally unrealistic.

"Jen, do you have to make dinner now?" Liza would say.

"The kids haven't eaten since noon; it's seven-thirty." She didn't understand the demands of motherhood.

After we exhausted the videos we had brought, Kodie and Austin were arguing over toys. Alexis and Devan are big girls and were bored, the younger children were getting on their nerves as well. Stephen was my savior. He assumed the majority of the responsibility for entertaining them with the exception of the six hours he found to play golf with David's friend. I'm sure he wouldn't call this time a vacation. We had absolutely no time together during the day and Austin insisted on sleeping on a mattress on the floor beside us; that plus my constant physical discomfort put us under pressure.

As we went upstairs to shower before the guests arrived, I asked Liza: "Do you feel like you are celebrating your child? You are going to be a mommy."

"It's like a dream. I'm going through the motions. I know it's my baby but it doesn't seem real. I see the waiting nursery and I see you pregnant. I feel like an onlooker," she confessed.

"La, this is a lesson in not having expectations. The reality will come to you when it does, in ways you could never predict. Be open, and don't let my big body take the meaning of the party away from you. This is your party, for you and your baby. Let's enjoy it." I told her these things hoping she would understand that I recognized the singular positions we were each in.

Soon, the shower was in full swing. The weather was clear and very hot. At least forty women arrived, some with their husbands; they were mostly friends of Liza and David. Aunt Suzy was there, of course, and Joe, Greg, and Max arrived with Stuart and Sophia and my friend Rachel, from high school in New York, and her mother, which gave me a sense of familiarity. My father was unable to come. Stanley came with his wife, Vivian, who acted like an out-of-place guest; they kept themselves apart, which was an additional knife to me. I felt lonely. I was desperately missing belonging to someone, and yet I belonged to my husband and my children. Aunt Suzy attempted to make me feel cherished. I missed my mother's being there in body to share this with me.

I'm not sure if Liza and David could focus on the reality of the baby's arrival in spite of the adorable gifts. I felt as though, with my presence, she was unable to coo or express real emotion.

It never occurred to me that Liza would make a speech. I suppose I didn't expect any public recognition. Just before the opening of the gifts, though, she stood up to express her feelings. I immediately became ill at ease and aware that I should respond. Instead, I became fixated on Liza and her quite public show of emotion, which for me was a shock to see. The more she teared and trembled, the more I felt compelled to comfort her. Reaching for Liza distracted me from my own torrent of emotions. I discovered that Liza has fabulous friends—women who have depth and sincerity, who truly care for her and are trying to connect with her through this period of change. A few of them took time to reach out to me with an attempt to understand my motives and how I felt now. I was envious of Liza's relationships. Outside of Hilary and Liza, I haven't made time to develop a circle of people with whom I can share a mutual love and respect.

Liza's friend Bonni didn't come to the shower. She called to tell us her son had an earache and her husband was working and couldn't stay with him. I didn't believe her. Bonni and I contended for Liza's friendship at college when they were roommates and I was the outsider. I believe she still feels that hostility and for that reason stayed away.

In a different vein, Liza has an ex–college boyfriend with whom she's kept up a strong relationship and extended to include David. Steven Donziger is thirty-six years old, a lawyer, with dark, boyish good looks, and I found him very sexy. He has been aware of all the ups and downs in this journey with Liza. Although we went to school together for a short while at American University, I had no recollection of him nor he of me. He made a point of observing me throughout the party, as well as charming everyone else he came into contact with. As he approached me to talk, I felt myself become challenged, flirtatious, and acutely aware of being a woman, things I haven't felt since the beginning of this project. Feelings I have been robbed of by the drugs and pregnancy. Steven was insightful and told me that in the beginning he didn't understand our reasons for doing what we were doing, but after hearing Liza's narrative and meeting me, he had complete compassion and it was clear why Liza and I had grown spiritually during the process. It felt wonderful to be attracted to someone and play with the idea that he was attracted to me in spite of my huge pregnant body.

I was given some heartfelt gifts. An oil painting by Aunt Suzy of a little boy looking at a vase of flowers will hang in the entrance hall of our house. Liza gave me an equipped gym bag and health-club membership. I guess my size impressed her.

After everyone left, Greg, Max, and Rachel, Stephen and I, David and Liza were left to discuss the day and hang out. I was overtired at this point. My feet were swollen, so that the skin at the base of my toes split and my legs were swollen. I took my shoes off and lay down on the porch. Stephen came quickly to my aid, as usual, with a huge commercial bag of ice, and Liza brought me a wet washcloth. I was in agony; even so, it was nice to talk and compare notes about the shower.

We talked about how we missed Jack, who couldn't come because he was doing a music job for a club in Montauk, and Erica, who couldn't come for another unlikely reason. This prefaced the one event of the day I found most distressing. We began to talk about the baby.

Greg and Max expressed their joy for Liza and David, but as parents for eight years, they were, I think, quick to dole out unsolicited advice. A conversation about physicians and inoculations arose. Max jumped in as an expert on the risks involved in each of the recommended inoculations. Hearing Maxine tell Liza, with absolute certainty, which shots the baby should receive and which he should not, was more than I could bear. My reaction was pretty strong. I excused myself, not being able to sit there and listen to what Max wanted done with a child that was growing inside my body, that I had nurtured and loved and would have to relinquish care of. In my head I was prepared for Liza and David to make the decisions that would affect his life, but not Max, who had done nothing to bring this baby into the world.

My sense of ownership of the baby took me over without warning and it frightened me greatly. I went upstairs and cried, realizing that soon I will not be the one supervising the care of this child; this awareness was not as clear-cut as I had thought it would be. I hope it won't develop into an ongoing struggle.

The day, in total, was distressing. I wanted it to be Liza's day and a celebration of our love. It took on a much deeper significance.

The days that followed seemed endless; each of us had encased ourselves in an impenetrable sheath of protection. We became two embittered camps. We left in a mockery of sad good-byes.

Soon after I was at home in Chicago, Liza and I spoke of all the unexpressed feelings we'd had and didn't understand. Each of us was hurt by herself and by the other.

I apologized to Liza for my reaction to Maxine, and wrote Max a note saying so. Liza and I told each other what we had been experiencing. "Liza, I was so uncomfortable. It was so hot and I'm so big and I did feel out of place. My mother wasn't there and everyone else was so thin and beautiful. I was feeling sorry for myself. Not for the pregnancy, just . . . well, I went backward and then I was embarrassed in front of you, so I couldn't talk about it."

"I should have cornered you and gotten you alone. We would have ironed it out eventually. I was upset, too. We weren't being honest with each other."

"Honesty is so hard, first to yourself and then to admit it. Liza, I was being possessive of Luc: that's the honest truth. I felt if he isn't mine to rear, he certainly isn't in the realm of anyone else's advice."

"I was feeling guilty again," Liza said. "It was the first time *in a long time. I felt that guilt, but you were so miserable and you wouldn't let me help you."*

"And I really messed up your party. La. The party was for you and I made a spectacle of myself. I wanted this baby shower to be full of happiness and excitement for you."

"We were butting heads, me with guilt—"

"And me with jealousy. I feel better now that we talked it out. Do you?"

"Yes . . . yes. I do, Jen. I couldn't stand this between us. I knew all along I wouldn't see you until the birth. That will be the most intimate time, to see the baby we made be born. I want only love between us and nothing, nothing to mar that. Nothing will, no matter what. We have love, but it should be free of ill feelings. It will be. My God. I feel happy."

I have recorded this conversation in my journal to remember the sincerity of the words and how openly they were expressed.

September 2, 1997

Every morning I wake up afraid of what is ahead of me. I have nightmares about not being able to deliver the baby because of a cold or other complications. I am anxious to be done with the pregnancy, which has been my overpowering concern, and to get back to the folds of my own life and family.

As I approach the end of this journey, I concentrate on its purpose to heal me and teach me to let go of control, but I fear I am sliding backward and hope I will have strength to let go of Luc.

After my mother died, I prayed for the hurt, that was a raw slice through my heart, to be over. It is different now. I pray that I will be as strong as I tell myself I am. I have so much waiting for me. I have my husband, children, my father, and Hilary. People I couldn't hear after my mother's death.

I know I will make it through. I keep looking at my priorities and let the big picture fade in. I was blindly focusing on keeping my mother alive without allowing myself to see anything else. Now I will face life head-on and let it take its own course.

Six weeks. I have to stop myself from counting the days or trying to schedule the birth. Liza is also apprehensive. After the failure of our fantasy vacation, we are both aware of all that is at stake, not only through the birth but for the rest of our lives. We have promised to communicate so after Luc is born we will emerge healthy, independent, and loving. I have no regrets. People ask me if I think this is a path more women should take. This is much harder than words can express and I know that each person would have her own reasons: it is a question I can't answer for anyone else.

September 15, 1997

I fainted this weekend. Luckily I injured my pride, not the baby. We had been on the go all weekend, starting with a business dinner on Friday for Stephen. Saturday we took the kids to an amusement park and Sunday evening Ralph [Stephen's father] came to our house for the traditional family dinner, and to spend time with his grandchildren. Long periods of standing on my feet got the better of me, and I realized it was time to give in to daily naps.

Liza met with Arlene for three hours on Thursday while Arlene was in New York. I am so appreciative of the concern and interest she has shown to all of us through this process. More importantly, I have never known Liza to be forthright to a therapist, let alone voluntarily spend so much time with one. Liza said Arlene helped her through some of the mystery and difficulty she was facing about the actual birthing.

She was feeling guilty that she would be experiencing joy while I was in pain. Arlene suggested that she not dwell on my physical pain but be encouraging and supportive, and that we both should be prepared for unexpected feelings to arise. We must focus on the incredible bond we share. I do hope Arlene's support will help Liza and me communicate better.

October 5, 1997

I am anticipating Liza and David's arrival. Each night at eight o'clock Chicago time I begin to panic. That is the last scheduled flight from New York until six o'clock the next morning. If I should go into labor, I won't be able to reach Liza.

*J*ennifer was dilated 2 cm. Her mucus plug came out on Friday. On October 5, David and I stayed close to the phone and were prepared to rush to La Guardia Airport at a moment's notice. We didn't know exactly when to go. Dr. Isola said the baby still could take up to two weeks to arrive. We didn't want to risk not being there for the birth, but we also didn't want to hang around nervously waiting for two weeks. If David took time off now, he wouldn't be able to take it later. Plus, we worried about being in Jennifer's way at home. Our waiting around would make her nervous, and give her added work.

Our bags were packed. Luc's nursery was ready. Jennifer would tell us when to come.

Jennifer sounded calm, but I knew she was masking her anxiety. She was very active, hoping to bring on the labor. Dr. Isola said if nothing happened by the sixteenth, she would induce labor. So Luc would not be born on Jennifer's birthday—the nineteenth—after all. I was glad. They each deserved their own special day.

We had made a final decision on Luc's full name—Luc Alexander Freilicher, Alexander for David's maternal grandmother. It is a long name; the initials are L.A.F. I liked that.

It was unbelievable to me that we were at the final countdown.

The time had passed quickly, but when I remembered the years of heartbreaking disappointment, it seemed I had waited a lifetime for Luc. Any day, my life would change forever. How lucky we were, that someone was doing this incredible thing for us—bringing David and me a new life, making us a family.

On Thursday, October 9, I was on the plane to Chicago. David had to stay in New York to finish a presentation for one of his accounts. He planned to join me as soon as we had some news, or by Saturday, at the latest.

Stephen and Jen picked me up at the airport. I had wondered if any of the strain from our "vacation" would still linger despite the phone calls and airing of our feelings. Seeing her glowing face and sharing one hug erased all my concern.

Oh my! She was so beautiful, smiling as she carried Luc with great pride, and we hugged and kissed before I got in the backseat and we drove to Dr. Isola's office for what would be her last exam until the birth.

During the pregnancy, she had gained about forty-five pounds. That was a sacrifice. I knew she would get back into shape, but it would be a challenge. Surely, she had the motivation and I didn't doubt that she had the fortitude.

Chicago was the place where my baby had lived for nine months. Soon it would be time to bring him to New York, and he would be mine. I couldn't wait to hold Luc.

October 11, Saturday

Over the past two days of waiting, Liza and I have vigorously walked around the neighborhood, hoping the exercise would encourage Luc to greet the world. Kodie enjoyed coming with us and talked about the baby. Austin stayed home under Christine's watchful eye. At night I spent time alone with Kodie, helping with homework while Liza played with Austin. It is good that Liza is here with us so the children can visibly understand that she is Luc's mother and is here for his birth—

that it is okay for both of us. They are excited to meet their cousin. This time between La and me is easy. Liza went to the market for me and put the groceries away while I watched from the kitchen table telling her where everything went. After, she delightedly made lunch for us. I was enjoying myself. Why had we ruined what could have been the same pleasant time at her house? I suppose it was a learning period and now we have discarded all that baggage of unresolved childhood problems. Whatever it was, it is behind us and we are peaceful in our hearts.

Now that she is here I don't feel any tension about what is coming. It has been hard to wait for a baby that is not mine. If hormones don't rise up and make my emotions run amok, I should be fine. I can't wait to see Liza's face at the birth and to share with her the exaltation—all that we have dreamed and schemed for.

I keep hoping that Luc will come before the inducement on Thursday. I enjoy the thrill of dashing to the hospital and the nervousness of labor. I want Liza to experience that part of the pregnancy.

David arrived last night and we buzzed around all morning getting my things, Liza's things, and Luc's necessities ready for the hospital.

October 13, 1997

It's Columbus Day and three days prior to the scheduled inducement on the sixteenth. The family is beginning to arrive. My father is here, so are Alexis and Devan, who are sleeping downstairs in the playroom. Every bed and sofa in the house is occupied. Hilary is on alert.

I realize Liza and David won't be coming back to the house on Friday from the hospital. I know this is the best thing. We all need space and distance to make adjustments, but for me, loneliness is beginning to emerge. I miss my mother, and though I have an army of people as a safety net around me, I'm afraid. I am crying tears I've held in for a long time. The moment I've thought of and idealized is almost upon me— handing the baby to Liza and seeing the rapture in her face. Right now I can't feel it. Right now I am terrified.

October 14, 1997

Today doesn't seem as overwhelming as yesterday. Last night I could hardly breathe with the torment of separation I was feeling. I was in my room just for some quiet time and to get away from watchful eyes. I called down for Stephen to come upstairs.

"Hold me. Hold me. I don't think I can do this," I cried, and clung to him. It must have been a measure of my doubt that I had no shame in showing my weakness. He held me.

"Jen, you're going to be all right, and when it's over you will be all you planned on becoming. We will be together. Can Liza come up to sit with you? She asked me if it would be all right."

I nodded and smiled. I was feeling comforted. It was actually better for me to be with Liza, just the two of us, together. We reminisced about long-past memories, reestablishing the solidarity of our early lives.

"Jen . . ." Liza said very seriously, looking down and fingering the edge of the pillowcase. "I have a confession."

I didn't know what to brace myself for. "A confession?"

She nodded. "I ate the chocolate pudding."

"Aha!" I whooped. "I knew it. All these years. It was you. You sneak!"

"Remember we were having a sleepover at my house—"

"And your mother made a chocolate pudding which she left in cups on the kitchen table to cool overnight."

"Well . . . I woke up early. You were asleep, so I went downstairs to get the comic books we'd left in the kitchen. I

saw the pudding. I was hungry. I ate it and put the dish in the sink."

"When she asked, 'How was the chocolate pudding? Who ate it?' . . . why didn't you admit it?"

"I don't know."

"And all the while she knew it was one of us."

"Or it could have been my father. He loves chocolate."

"I wish I'd thought of that. It would have been a good opportunity to get him back for all the times he yelled at me for eating the frosting off cakes."

"I thought of that."

We laughed so hard, spit spattered from our mouths.

"It was a fun mystery," Liza stated.

"Who ate the chocolate pudding?" we chimed together.

"Does your mother know?"

"Nope. I played it cool," she said in triumph. "I was in control. Every birthday my mother asked who ate the pudding and I never flinched. I'll tell her next time she asks. Do you have any confessions?"

I thought awhile "Well . . . as a matter of fact . . . I borrowed your red sweater."

"Borrowed? I never got it back."

"I forgot. Then I was scared." I looked at her sheepishly.

The door opened and Stephen put his head in and wryly asked, "What's all the noise?"

"Nothing," we replied slyly, and burst out laughing as he closed the door.

I still didn't tell Liza how terrified I was about the birth. It would hurt her deeply. She was afraid for my suffering and so ready to assume guilt. I was frightened because this was the culmination of all our research and work and creation. I was frightened as a well-rehearsed actor is before the curtain goes up. I have the starring role until Luc enters. Self-doubt, I believe is a human frailty. I knew how I felt psychologically, and emotionally I'd gotten myself straight. I prayed I would play my part well.

Hilary called me first thing this morning to check up on me and see how my night went. Everyone is looking at me. I feel as though I am having to entertain them.

We are two days from the birth. I keep hoping Luc will arrive early. Unfortunately I feel absolutely fine, with no signs of labor. I wait for Liza to experience the fun of "hurry, the baby is coming. Hurry!" In two days I will feel empty. I pray that the joy of Liza and David will overcome my fear and emptiness.

It was the day before Dr. Isola would induce labor if Jennifer didn't go into it on her own. We kept going. Jennifer sent David out to the store to buy a bag of potatoes and baby formula. He couldn't find the formula in the local pharmacy, so he drove a few miles farther away to find it. He came back much later with the formula and the potatoes. I had been anxious. As always I thought something awful might have happened, just as I worry about Jennifer or my mother, or Greg, Stuart, Sophia, and Max when they are out of touch or not where I expect them to be. This was my vulnerability. I supposed it related to my mother's accident, that day when devastation struck so suddenly while I was feeling protected and secure, surrounded by a happy active family. Tragedy overturned my life in an instant. That such an event would happen again was a dread that clutched my heart, especially in times of merriment.

The high-wired tension was on. We were camped in the Scheu living room after dinner. No one had eaten much. While the television was blaring no one was watching. We were each wrapped in our own thoughts. Each was concerned for the other.

I looked at the little empty bassinet next to me and knew it would soon have my baby son in it. "Please let him be well, healthy, and happy"—my constant prayer. "Please let Jen have an easy time of it: the birth and the time after. Let her be fulfilled by this incredible act, free of pain and suffering." I knew this would take time, but I prayed that it would come sooner rather than later and that her wondrous gift would give her the happiness she was seeking in her own life. The following day would be Luc's birthday. "Please let that date be one we'll always celebrate together—celebrate the birth of our baby and the rebirth of Jennifer's life. Let it be the day we will especially thank Aunt Laurie. She is with all of us to-night. She is watching over us, as my mother is. The union of four persevering women, powered by love and clear intent, is solid and strong. Let tomorrow be a day of tears, but tears of happiness and miracles, joy and excitement, and anticipation of a happy, long life together—a life as a family: Liza, David, and Luc. See you tomor-row, my baby."

Ralph, Stephen's father, called late that night. The sudden ringing startled us. As I feared, the peace was interrupted. According to Ralph, someone from the hospital called the Illinois Department of Health wanting to check on the order that the judge had sent there stating that David and Liza Freilicher were the legal and natural parents of the child to be delivered by Jennifer Scheu. This order had never been presented to the hospital before. And, of course, some unnamed clerk, having no legal background, told them that despite any court order they had, this unorthodox arrangement was not acceptable. This, on the night before the baby would be born! Panic set in. Was I going to have to go through the procedure of adopting my baby after all? Was the court order meaningless? Ralph would let us know as soon as he could. "I'm working on it," he said.

"My father is unstoppable," Stephen said in full faith. "He'll pull us through."

With that, we all went to our beds, trying to prepare for the birth and the baby. Neither David nor I slept and I'm sure Jenni-fer and Stephen didn't either. If there was to be an adoption it would be a long-drawn-out venture that would require all of us to be present in court, Jennifer weak from delivery and me with a newborn infant.

I lay in bed that night looking at the ceiling. I must have spent hours like that. I thought of the long-ago times when Jennifer and I skipped from rock to rock along a running stream. Jennifer's greatest fear had been to be separated from her mother. Tomorrow, she prayed, she would be released from that pain. My greatest fear was devastation from the unexpected. Here, today, so many years and experiences later, we were on the brink of facing our own terrors head-on.

Chapter
48

*D*avid and I got up at five in the morning. It was dark outside. We dressed quickly. I wore black slacks and a white T-shirt, a brown cardigan sweater, brown socks and shoes, and a black blazer. My hair was clean and straight, since I'd borrowed Jen's blow-dryer.

We had breakfast in the kitchen and took pictures of each other, surrounded with the paraphernalia we were bringing to the hospital. We were tired but smiling.

Jen took my hand as we went outside to leave, placing her other hand on her belly. She was smiling. "I won't hold him like this again. I know he is a wonderful baby, Liza. I love him. I've taken good care of him for you. I know you will be a wonderful mother. He knows you. He knows your voice and off-key singing." She laughed and then put her arms around me and cried softly. I, too, cried for the beauty of it all and for the emotions for which there are no words.

The moon was full. David and I took Stephen's car. The rest of them went in Jen's Toyota van.

It was 6:30 A.M. when we checked into the hospital. Ralph left us a message that he had scheduled a meeting with one of the associate general counsels for the hospital later that morning and would make sure we received word of the results of this meeting even if we were in the birthing room. But we could not think about the legal problem now.

All of us—imagine the crowd—walked into the birthing room. It was bright and large and, surprisingly, bore no resemblance to an operating room. We had a private bathroom equipped with tooth-paste and smelling salts, which I knew I would not need.

We met Leanne, our nurse. She smiled sweetly and I could tell immediately that she had a calming influence on Jen, who went into the bathroom to put on the gown she had been given.

Hilary, Jen's father, Martin, David, Stephen, and I sat quietly, preparing our cameras, and soon Jen returned from the bathroom. Leanne helped her into the bed. "Are you feeling any contractions?" she asked.

Jennifer shook her head no, and lay back.

Leanne cranked up the bed so Jen's legs were bent and her head was raised to survey the audience, then Leanne started an intrave-nous drip of the medication that would induce labor. She said, as she inserted the needle into Jennifer's vein, that she couldn't deal with having her own blood drawn but considered herself an expert with IVs. She and Jen were joking with each other, trying to keep the mood light.

Leanne explained the operation of the fetal monitor and machine that notes all the contractions. She hooked Jen up to these two ma-chines with a belt across her belly.

Just then there was a knock at the door. I opened it. "Is this Scheu/Freilicher?" said a young man in a white staff jacket. His ID read CLERICAL DEPARTMENT.

"Yes," I said, my heart beating. He handed me an envelope. I knew it was the results of Ralph's meeting. I closed the door and handed the envelope to David. My hands were damp. I was afraid to open it.

David opened the envelope and glanced at the bottom of the page quickly. His face broke into a huge smile. "Ralph did it," he an-nounced so loudly that Leanne said "shh."

David and I embraced. He wiped the tear that was coursing down my cheek. "That's all settled, Luc will be born Freilicher." He handed me a tissue to blow my nose, and I gave Jennifer a high five.

"Couldn't you have had a better last name?" I joked to David.

He mockingly punched me in the arm.

Jennifer looked up at me and smiled. "I'm eager to start labor, to have Luc here for you, and to get my life back. I have a husband waiting for me." She took Stephen's hand.

I pushed the hair back from her forehead. She looked so glamorous, as if she were going to a party with her hair up in a French knot.

She flinched and I saw on the screen that the first contraction had begun.

"La, it's starting. I'm familiar with birthing. I don't want you to be disgusted or uncomfortable with David here watching me have a baby. I don't want you to feel as if I'm taking your place." She spoke so no one heard us. As if no one else were in the room.

I kissed her head. "Don't worry about me. To see you give birth to our son will be the most memorable, beautiful experience of our lives."

After an hour, when the contractions were coming stronger and with shorter intervals, Dr. Isola came in and told me to stand by Jennifer's feet to watch the birth. I was reluctant to leave Jennifer's side. Hilary stood in my place and patted Jen's head, reminding her to keep breathing and helping her get through the contractions.

At 9:15 A.M. Jennifer asked to get an epidural injection to numb the pain. She was 4 cm. dilated.

We left the room as the anesthesiologist prepared the syringe.

I felt awful waiting outside, knowing Jen was getting that injection in her spine. I had seen it done in a Lamaze video and it had frightened me. Again I was struck by Jennifer's bravery.

When we were called back into the birthing room, Jen's father was asked to wait outside. Jennifer said she was okay, but there were beads of perspiration on her head and she was biting her lip.

I expected to be overwhelmed by the doctors, Jen's pain, and the lack of privacy Jennifer submitted to, but I didn't feel anxious, I was excited.

We waited. Jen was uncomfortable even though the epidural was taking effect. She was nauseous and threw up several times as a result of the medications.

At eleven-forty-five, a nurse examined Jennifer and said she was 7 cm. dilated and that it shouldn't be much longer. She went to find Dr. Isola.

I held David's hand.

Jen said she felt like she had to push. Leanne told her to try not to, to wait for the doctor.

Dr. Isola finally arrived. I could see the relief in Jennifer's face.

We took our designated positions. Jen put her feet in the stirrups. Hilary stood by her head. David was by her right knee holding her leg; Leanne was holding her left knee. Dr. Isola was between her legs. I was next to the doctor by her right leg, next to David, who was weeping openly—from the release of anxiety and the exhilaration of this very long-awaited moment, the birth of his son, the answer to his prayers. At Jennifer's request, Stephen was filming it all on his video camera.

"Do you want to help deliver your son?" Dr. Isola asked me.

"Yes." I put on a gown, slippers, and tight latex gloves. I was nervous.

Jennifer was lying back, feeling dizzy. The drugs made her eyeballs slide from side to side. At Dr. Isola's instructions, she began to push. Hilary stood by her, stroking her head and instructing her on when to breathe. I watched as her body swelled, and slowly expanded.

At noon, I saw the baby's head as he crowned through the birth canal. He looked tiny. Too tiny? The doctor kept touching Jennifer, stretching the opening. Jen was crying out. Her cries cut me to the heart.

We watched Luc's head appear and disappear for several minutes. I could not imagine how a baby could survive such a tight squeeze.

Dr. Isola made a small incision in the bottom of the birth canal so Luc's head and shoulders could pass without ripping the delicate tissue there.

"You're doing fine, Jennifer," she said encouragingly.

Little by little my baby's head emerged. I watched in complete fascination . . . my baby was being born.

The doctor told me to take a position on Jen's right side so I would be able to help. Luc's head was out. "Put your hand on his neck and then ease him upward."

Dr. Isola had one hand and I had both hands on Luc. At 12:16 P.M. he slid out easily and immediately was howling. A team cheer went up from everyone in the room. Jen was intently watching my face.

All of a sudden he was here. "Oh my God . . . thank God," I breathed, not knowing if my words were audible.

He was covered in a cheesy white film. All I could see was his back. I didn't see his face.

The doctor laid him on Jen's chest. She had her hands on him. I was frustrated; everyone could see him but me. When the doctor summoned me, I ran to Jen's side so I could see his face.

Oh, he was strong, he had a scrunched-up little face and long dark hair. He was yelling. He was perfect.

I couldn't take my eyes off him. Today was the day he was mine. I looked at all his parts. He was no longer a dream.

David cut the umbilical cord. It happened so fast, I didn't even see him do it. I was counting toes and fingers, marveling at this creation. Dr. Isola brought him to an examining table under a heat lamp. He was screaming hardily and soon his skin was rosy. I cut the umbilical cord shorter where the doctor indicated; she put a clip on it. Luc was given an identification bracelet: Luc Alexander Freilicher, a long name for such a tiny wrist. And I was given a bracelet, too, identifying me as Luc Freilicher's mother.

The hospital pediatrician checked Luc and reported that we had a perfect baby boy, eight pounds, two ounces, strong and healthy. He was footprinted. And Leanne said she would bring each of us a T-shirt with his footprints on it before we left the hospital. Luc was cleaned and swaddled in a blue receiving blanket and cap and given to his mother: *me*.

One minute he wasn't here and the next he was a person in the world, documented by his footprints. "He is here. Luc is here. He is my baby. Now he belongs wholly to David and me. I can't believe it . . . I can't believe it. Jen, look what we did!"

Jennifer's face was shining through her tears of joy. "It happened.

We did it." Her voice was strong—absolute and sure as she had been from the start.

I just wanted to look at him and touch him all over to learn his feel, make sure he was fine, keep my eyes on him. I couldn't take my eyes from my baby, my son. Immediately I was his guardian, his protector. I was his mommy.

When Dr. Isola placed him in my arms, it felt so natural, so different from holding someone else's child. He was mine.

David held him next. He was so overwhelmed he didn't know what to do with himself. He just cried, which he does only when he can't express himself.

I really knew Jennifer was very uncomfortable. She had to be sewed up and was still feeling nausated from the medicine. She held the baby with love. She looked at me and we hugged each other and cried wordlessly with Luc in both our hands. I didn't know what to do with my immense gratitude.

I picked him up and sat in a chair. The rest of the room dissolved from my sight. I only had eyes for my son.

"I have to call Aunt Suzy. La, I'm calling your mother," Jennifer said as Hilary helped her sit up and brought her a lipstick. She was the most radiant of all of us. So proud of herself. I heard Jennifer talking to my mother.

"You should see your daughter, Aunt Suzy. She's holding her son and beaming. We did it, all of us. Mommy was right. Oh, my God I'm looking at them."

I couldn't hear my mother. But Jennifer said, "I feel great. I can't wait to get to the gym." She paused. "Don't cry, we are all laughing. I'll send you the tape so you can see everything, his entire birth . . . Yes, we taped it. I love you, too. Congratulations, Grandma."

She passed me the phone. "Ma, he's here, he is so beautiful, I can't believe it. Jen did such an incredible job, I can't believe I'm holding my baby. It feels so great, so right." I told her I would call her back in a little while once we all got settled, and passed the phone to David.

I had asked my mother to join us in Chicago, but she felt she would be too much of a responsibility for me and did not want to distract us. "I'll be there in spirit with my sister," she had told me.

David held Luc and called his parents. Stephen and Hilary were caring for Jen and continued to take pictures. We moved from the birthing room to the hospital room. Jen held Luc while they wheeled her down the hall. It was hospital regulations. "La, I'm sorry. I hope this doesn't bother you. We didn't think of this."

"No." I laughed. "It doesn't bother me." And truly, it didn't.

Jennifer was tired but feeling better. Ralph came and brought Kodie and Austin. We thanked him and told him he was a step-grandfather, and the children each sat in a chair and held Luc. I was surprised at myself, how calm I was. They looked at their new cousin in awe and Luc made sweet baby noises. Toward evening, the visitors began to leave, Hilary first, and then Stephen took Kodie and Austin home. Then it was just Jen, David, me, and Luc, looking incredulously at one another. The future was all before us.

We ordered dinner, which took forever. Luc slept most of the time. Jen was feeling better. The tension dissipated.

Later, after David had returned to the hotel, I made up the small bed the hospital had provided for me. Jen was tired and soon fell asleep. I was glad she could finally rest. I didn't want to take my eyes off Luc. I moved the bassinet next to my cot and just stared at him. After a couple of hours, I felt myself begin to doze. I was nervous about leaving my baby unsupervised, so I brought him to the nursery. One nurse was tough looking, with long dreadlocks and wicked-looking fingernails, a ring on each finger. She didn't appear "nursish" to me, and I didn't feel safe leaving my baby with her. But then another nurse, a quiet, neat, and gentle-looking one appeared. I stayed in the nursery for an hour. I'm sure they didn't approve of that.

The nurse with dreadlocks looked at me questioningly, wondering how I could possibly be the mother. The other nurse said to me, "Why don't you get some sleep?"

Obviously, all other mothers were too exhausted to sit in the nursery at three A.M.

Eventually, and reluctantly, I went back to the room and slept for a while. I couldn't believe I had my own darling baby.

I woke at five A.M. to check on Luc in the nursery. He was asleep. Such a good baby. I brought him back to the room with a bottle of formula and tried not to wake Jen. I just stared at them both in amazement.

Chapter

49

Jennifer opened her eyes from sleep to see me giving Luc his bottle. She stretched and winced at the soreness she felt in her body, then her face broke into a wide smile. Her eyes were bright.

"I love those little purring sounds he makes. Luc is a happy baby. Look at him take his bottle."

I brought him over and laid him on the bed in Jen's arms.

"He's a strong person, all the odds he overcame to be here. He doesn't even look like a newborn, La, he's pink and rosy, his face is smooth." She exclaimed, "What a beautiful, wondrous baby."

"You kept him that way," I said. "He's a happy baby. He didn't fuss last night." I watched Luc suck the bottle in Jen's arms, and wondered if she had the urge to nurse the infant she had birthed. Now that she could see that my goal had been reached, I wondered how close she was to attaining hers, but I knew that for now this was just idle speculation. It would take time.

She raised herself up in the bed and adjusted Luc on her shoulder to burp him. "Liza, I can't believe I am looking at our beautiful creation. My body is uncomfortable, but I am so happy he is here."

Dr. Isola entered the room as Jen was handing Luc to me. She peered into the bunting. His baby mouth was puckered, looking for a nipple. He opened his eyes and looked at his mommy. He was warm and his baby hair smelled like fresh grass to me as I kissed the top of his head.

Dr. Isola signed Jen's release and we were ready to leave the hospital. "I will always remember this baby," the doctor said, smiling. "They say that all men are created equal, but it's not true for Luc. He struggled harder to get here and he has come bravely into a world with so much love." She kissed Jen on the forehead.

David and Stephen arrived soon after Jennifer was dressed. She was made up and sitting in nonmaternity clothes, impatient to go home and be with Kodie and Austin. Of course she had left her trousers unbuttoned and her long jacket open over her spread hips. But looking at Jen, no one would have guessed she had just given birth. It took some time to get Luc ready for his first outing, but finally we were on our way out of the hospital.

A nurse escorted all of us downstairs, Jen had to be in a wheelchair, hospital policy. When we reached the lobby, the men went for the cars. Jen slowly got up. She was wearing her high heels and stood tall. To me she was heads and shoulders above anyone on earth.

Hilary met us in the lobby and I could see how delighted Jen was to see her.

David was having trouble strapping down the car seat. "I'll do it," I said.

"Liza, look, it's done."

"We're going to leave you to figure this out for yourselves," Jennifer announced. "We'll see you at the house tomorrow. I won't call you."

This time Jennifer was leaving without Luc. I thought of all the times during the months he was growing and living inside of her when I'd fly off to New York, leaving her in Chicago, and leaving my baby with her. It had been painful. Now at last it was me leaving with Luc. I hoped this separation wouldn't cause her to suffer. I hoped she would achieve her goal.

I sat in the backseat next to Luc. David drove carefully to the hotel. We were on our own for the rest of our lives.

October 17, 1997

When the car pulled away from the hospital leaving Liza and David with Luc, separating us for the first time, I truly missed him. I felt empty. We drove in silence. Both Hilary and Stephen respected my private time with my thoughts. During the last month I had been afraid I wouldn't survive giving up the baby I was carrying, to whom I have been relating and whom I love. Not because I felt he was my own but because of the interrelationship and sense of dependency we have shared, he depending on me for life and me depending on him to fill the void of my loneliness. I sought my soul, sitting next to my husband, looking at him in silence, looking out the window at life around me. Yes, I was happy and I was glad. I knew I had been awakened to the love my mother had given to me. I wanted Stephen to drive quickly so I could be home with my children. I opened the window and closed my eyes, letting the breeze blow on my face. The air was fragrant as it filled my lungs. I breathed deeply. That scent? The familiar scent, the sign I had been waiting for. My mother's covenant, our pact. I breathed deeply the sheltering warmth of my mother. There was no doubt. I opened my eyes and looked at Stephen. He appeared not to have noticed. I closed my eyes again in peace, secure in the knowledge that I would survive without my mother and without the baby next to me. I was whole without them here to make me special. Today I am Jennifer Scheu, not only Laurie's daughter. I am strong enough to survive well.

David and I spent the rest of the day and night in the hotel room with our son, away from the world. No one called us and no one came to visit. Being a mother came so naturally to me—all the years I doubted myself, felt intruded upon by children, all the years I didn't understand Rafael's love and dedication to his sons . . . they all fell away. I was thrilled to be a mother. I was ready to give maternal love. I wasn't nervous giving Luc his bottle or changing him. David, too, handled him like he'd been a daddy forever.

We arrived at Jennifer's at ten for breakfast. She was up and about already, and enjoying a long-awaited cup of coffee. Jen was anxious to hear about Luc's night. Martin, Hilary, and the kids were taking turns holding him. Luc allowed himself to be passed around without a whimper. Jen gave him a bottle and changed his diaper, marveling at him and enjoying him so. When I asked her how she was feeling, she said, "Fine. If hormones don't mess me up, I'm fine, La. It was a worthwhile trip. The medicine was often hard to take, but the cure was worth it."

As one o'clock approached, we had to prepare to leave for the airport. I had a lump in my throat. I knew we were feeling emotional and anxious. David started to pack up the car, and I put Luc in his bunting.

Jen got up to walk us out.

We embraced. After a couple of minutes, Kodie, too, came over; she touched Luc's hand. We were awash in tears and smiles. There were no words for this farewell.

October 19, 1997

Today is my birthday. I'm glad the birth is over and I have my day all to myself, which I spent the best way possible—at home with my husband and my children. Stephen grilled steaks; he and Kodie cleaned the kitchen while Austin and I lay in our big bed together waiting for them to come upstairs and watch The Little Mermaid *for the third time.*

Liza called to wish me happy birthday and Luc made precious noises. It was a most happy birthday. And I felt my mother's joyful presence.

Chapter
50

At twenty-two days old, Luc already seemed to be outgrowing his infancy. We had his bris at our apartment, which was not pleasant, but we got through it. Jennifer preferred to remain in Chicago. She wanted this time to be for Luc and his parents without upstaging us by having to answer questions. I hadn't gone back to work. I spent almost every minute with Luc, getting to know him.

I felt his presence in my life and in my heart. I knew every inch of him, his every need and desire, each whimper. I looked into his eyes and he into mine and he knew me as well as if he'd grown in my womb. He responded to my voice. I was awed by how a mother animal, for that was what I was, knows her own, how her heart beats for and her senses are acutely attuned to her offspring. To know Luc was to at last know myself fully. And I knew why parents only have this kind of love for their children, why Jennifer felt Luc was not her child, and how she was able to separate from him.

The weather in New York had been unseasonably warm due to the phenomenon of "El Niño," making it possible for me and Luc to spend time outside.

We walked through the park many times. I was happy to be part

of the women pushing baby carriages. Luc and I spent a lot of time
with my mother. She would meet us on her scooter, and we traveled
along Madison Avenue looking in windows. I don't know where the
hours of the day flew. I only know I wanted to be with Luc every
second. I just stared at him when he slept in his crib at night and
held him all day.

I had come to understand why Jennifer catered to her children
and how precious her time at home with them was to her. I also
sympathized with the way Rafael had made his boys his top priority.
I owed an apology to all the mothers and fathers whom I considered
shallow and unaccomplished because of their total absorption in
indulgence of their children. I sympathized painfully with my
mother, who suffered Erica's illness and torments. How my grandmother was able to survive her daughter's death seemed beyond
anything I ever wanted to imagine. I apologized for my closed mind,
but at the time, I had been blind. Surely, I had role models whom I
loved and respected: my mother and Aunt Laurie, whose children
were the preeminent beings in their lives. Jennifer told me, Bonni
told me, women of different temperament but with the same innate
maternal commitment. I hadn't understood. Perhaps because I
thought such feelings weren't part of my nature—I, who as a child,
hadn't even played with dolls. Looking back, I didn't recognize in
myself any of the maternal instincts I saw so clearly in Dakota—the
tender way she touched Luc's hand, and the way she looked out for
her younger brother, Austin.

I spoke to Jennifer each morning and each night. My mother also
talked to her daily and we conferred with each other to be certain
that she was doing well. She was working out at the gym and miraculously had lost most of the weight she'd gained during the pregnancy. One day, she announced triumphantly, "My waistline is
back!" I told her about Luc and our quiet days together. She felt
such pleasure when I told her of his slightest change and progress—
how he was eating, the hours he slept, how he looked at me.

I was confident that Jen had no regrets. She handled the separation smoothly and she wore her heroism well.

· · ·

The phone rang; it was Hanna, my neighbor.

"Are you busy?" she asked mysteriously.

"No, why?"

"Meet me at the door in three minutes," she told me.

Three minutes later, I opened the door to find Hanna holding her familiar light blue Tiffany bag, the one that had been filled with needles and syringes. I cringed at the memory.

"These are for you," she said.

I opened the bag to find tiny blue, yellow, and white baby footie pajamas.

I hugged Hanna. Both of us had tears in our eyes.

When Luc was two months old, Jennifer flew to New York for a short visit to see him. Not wanting to sleep in the nursery with Luc, she spent the night at her father's house and came over early in the morning so we'd have a full day together.

We spent the morning in the nursery. Jen watched me bathe Luc, and then she gave him his bottle while I made some business calls. It was so natural and relaxed, the three of us interacting. "Are you ever going back to work?" she asked.

"I've been going to the restaurant during the day and taking Luc with me. I know I'll soon have to get a baby-sitter so I can work part-time, but I keep putting it off, and truthfully, I resent the very idea," I told Jen.

During the afternoon, we took Luc for a short walk in the carriage. When the weather turned cold, we came home and I showed Jen all the gifts Luc had received and my photo album, which was already full of pictures.

There were pictures of Greg holding Luc at the bris.

"La, I hope you understand why I didn't come. I wanted it to be your day and I wanted to postpone my trip so we could spend the time together like we are instead of with a crowd and distractions."

"What a crazy day that was. I'm glad you weren't here."

I put Luc in his crib for his nap. When I came back to the living room, Jen was writing in her journal.

December 19, 1997

*This will be the last entry in this journal. I have found closure
to the sadness in my life. Perhaps I will start another journal
one day, but for now I am happy with my husband and my
children and not trying to solve any mysteries. My mother will
always be a part of my daily life. I have learned to live with
the pain of missing her. I don't want that pain to ever leave
me, but I look now beyond the pain and see myself as an adult,
fired from within by Mommy's love.*

By the time Luc woke from his nap and we had dressed and given
him a bottle, it was time to go across town to Greg's restaurant,
Bistro Le Steak. Jen and I were as close as ever. I felt no restraint
on my part or hers.

When Jennifer walked into the restaurant, all heads turned. Her
height, her way of carrying herself, and her long blond hair made it
impossible not to notice her. My mother hugged her. Jen took off
her black jacket and showed off her long-legged figure in black trousers and a low-cut black sweater.

We sat in the rear banquette and I put Luc in his infant seat next
to me. "Excuse me," I apologized to the two women at the next
table. They looked like mother and daughter. "I hope this won't
crowd you."

"Not at all." The older woman moved over.

"He's an adorable baby. How old is he?" asked the younger
woman.

"Two months," I replied proudly. The waiter took our drink order. Jennifer ordered white wine. So did I.

"How about champagne?" Mom asked.

"Champagne," David and Joe agreed, and continued the conversation they were having at the other side of the table.

The waiter popped the cork on a bottle of chilled Dom Pérignon
that Greg sent over from the bar.

"I love that sound," Jen said.

We toasted all around the table.

"To Jennifer," Mom said.

"To Liza."

"To Luc." David stood up.

"To all of us," Joe finished.

I handed Luc to Jen, saying to the ladies next to me, "I'm sorry to disturb you again."

They had finished their dinner and were paying their bill. "Congratulations to you all. Are you the mother?" the younger asked.

"Yes. I'm the mother; I'm Liza. This is my cousin Jennifer; she carried our baby for us. She gave birth to Luc," I said, happy to show Jen off.

"I'm Becky Platt. My mother . . . Naomi. I started IVF this month. You've given me such inspiration. We're lucky; today there are so many ways to put a family together."

Jen and I looked at each other and then at Becky Platt. Becky had a long road to travel. We didn't know her, but at once felt a connection. I could read in Jennifer's eyes and posture how proud she was of both of us. How spiritually lofty we both were. Becky looked at Luc as a realized dream. "My own baby becomes a possibility when I see how happy and successful you are. Thank you. Goodbye . . . Jennifer . . . Liza. Thank you very much."

She started away then turned and embraced each of us before rushing off. Jennifer and I were uncharacteristically silent, thinking of all we had been through. Luc was sleeping. David, Joe, and my mother were talking. And Jen and I were alone in the enormity of our deed.

"Liza, I have something for you," Jennifer said softly.

"I think you're given me enough, Jen."

"Close your eyes."

I put Luc in the infant seat and did as she requested. I felt Jennifer place something around my neck. I touched it, and knew at once what it was. I opened my eyes and saw the locket that my mother had given Aunt Laurie when Jennifer was born. The locket Laurie had given to Jennifer when Kodie was born. Jennifer had worn it to the hospital for our first consultation with Scot. Inside had been photos of Kodie and Austin.

I opened the locket. Inside was a picture of Luc.